THE WAY

origins of the mediterranean diet

DARIO GIUGLIANO
MICHAEL SEDGE - JOSEPH SEPE

THE WAY THEY ATE
origins of the mediterranean diet

G
IDELSON - GNOCCHI

THE WAY THEY ATE
origins of the mediterranean diet
D. Giugliano
M. Sedge - J. Sepe

© Idelson-Gnocchi Publishers,
12255 N.W. Hwy 225-A, Reddick, FL 32686 USA - Tel. (352) 591-1136 - Fax (352) 591-1189
E-mail: candotti@worldnet.net.att - http://www.idelson-gnocchi.com

DARIO GIUGLIANO, M.D., Ph.D.
Professor of Metabolic Diseases - Second University of Naples, Italy

MICHAEL SEDGE
Director-at-Large for the American Society of Journalists and Authors

JOSEPH SEPE, M.D.
Adjunct Professor - Life Sciences - University of Maryland University College

Contributors
Dr. CATERINA CICIRELLI, Soprintendenza Archeologica, Pompeii
Prof. PASQUA CICCARELLI, Istituto Superiore Educazione Fisica, Naples
GIOVANNI GIUGLIANO, student of medicine, Second University of Naples
FRANCESCO GIUGLIANO, student of medicine, Second University of Naples

Special thanks to all government agencies, institutions, libraries and others that contributed to this book. In particular, sincere gratification goes out to the Museo della Maschera, del Folklore e della Civiltà of Acerra and the Museo della Civiltà Contadina "Michele Russo" of Somma Vesuviana.

GG

© Gruppo Editoriale Idelson - Gnocchi - since 1908
80133 Napoli (Italia) - Via A. De Gasperi, 55
Tel. ++39081 5524733 pbx - Fax ++39081 5518295
E-mail: idelgno@tin.it   http://www.idelson-gnocchi.com

Index

Preface

Never before has human kind experienced such a rise in life expectancy. This is even more important when one considers that only a century ago the average life-span in Europe was 40 years. It was not very different from the Greeks of Pericles or the Romans, whose lifetimes spanned 20-30 years. Today, a woman in Spain can expect to live 81 years, a man more than 78 years. Individuals over 60 years of age currently number 580 million, 355 million of which reside in so-called "developing" nations. By the year 2020, the over-sixty population of the world will reach one billion, 700 million alone in developing countries. The research and medical efforts of the past century have led to a constant and progressive decrease in infectious disease mortality. At the same time, there has been an increase in cancer, cardiovascular, and other diseases commonly related to aging.

This apparent paradox between the increase in life expectancy and rise in degenerative diseases offers food for thought. When the human body is allowed to survive longer, by reducing infections, hunger, war, and natural disasters, new risk factors emerge. Take cardiovascular disease, for example. This is one of the major problems of contemporary public health. In Western countries, infarction, stroke, and peripheral artery disease represent the major causes of death. Globally, however, infectious and prenatal diseases are the number one killers. Be that as it may, things are changing. Even in developing countries, populations are aging; albeit in worse conditions than in industrialized nations.

Projections by the World Health Organization for the coming years do not offer much optimism: the first twenty years of the new millennium will be characterized by a true epidemic in cardiovascular diseases. Coronary artery disease, which held fifth place among major disabling diseases of the 1990s, will move to the number one position – a sad world record. The reason behind this shift is the change in lifestyle of contemporary human populations. These changes, which in themselves increase risk factors, added to the growing elderly population, will cause incidences of cardiovascular disease to skyrocket. At the same time, sedentary lives, lack of physical activity, improper diet, and cigarette smoking will cause a rise in obesity, diabetes, alterations in blood lipids, and arterial hypertension, all powerful cardiovascular risk factors. It is estimated that within the next 20 years, cigarette smoking will be the number one public health threat, killing more than eight million people around the world.

Even the Europeans are getting fat. Examining the list of "chubby" European nations, one finds Germany very close to America. Italy and England share second place, with 47.4 percent of the men and 32.3 percent of the women overweight. The level of obesity in Italy, according to recent figures, will soon reach five million, meaning that 10 percent of the population will be affected. These are alarming figures, and give justification to those desiring to include obesity in the list of the top five diseases of social significance. The American Heart Association has already indicated obesity as one of the primary, independent risk factors for cardiovascular disease. In the United States, however, the problem of obesity is far wider spread than in Europe. Imagine, for instance, that one airline is considering increasing the size of seats in their aircraft because a growing number of travelers cannot fit into those currently being used.

In addition to the availability of food and the reduction of physical activity, an individual's genes may contribute to morbidity. The Arizona Native Americans are a prime example. For centuries they have lived primarily as farmers, subject to periodic famine. The change from this ancient lifestyle to that of the fast-food, snack mentality of modern America has caused an explosion of diabetes and obesity. The problem is so dramatic that half of the Pima tribe over 35 years of age now suffers from both diseases. The hypothesis that a "thrifty gene" exists, is reinforced by the following evidence: historically, such a gene was needed to insure, in the persons that carried it, a major resistance against nutritional deficiency (cycle deficiency), mediating the reduction of energy consumed and the storage of excess food. In other words, when an individual was finally able to satisfy his hunger, all of the food consumed but not immediately required was deposited as fat. Carriers of this gene, in an environment of food abundance, as we have today, are prime candidates for obesity.

Throughout this book, I have attempted to convince readers that it is necessary to follow a balanced diet, in combination with a healthy lifestyle. Generally, these elements go hand-in-hand; those who eat properly frequently exercise, do not smoke, and make a conscious effort where health is concerned. This is the lifestyle we need to promote. The only way to prevent known as well as unseen risk factors, such as the inherent obesity gene, is through education both at school and home. Providing insight into the value of nutritional balance and fitness will insure us a healthy future. Even as a secondary prevention, in those that have already suffered some form of disease, proper dietary habits can do much.

The cornerstone for the Mediterranean diet, as we know it today, came from Crete. Despite the fact that the farmers of Crete argued with investigators that their diet was poor and lacking of meat. The islanders failed to realize at that time that it was the small consumption of meat, high intake of natural foods, and daily work in the fields that resulted in their excellent state of health. Even more ironic is the fact that the epidemiologists who discovered the full benefit of the diet of this Mediterranean people came from the Rockefeller Foundation. The Mediterranean, it seems, is filled with such paradoxes.

This book represents an enthusiastic adventure in time and space. For the most part, for those who have lived a part of their lives in a traditional farming environment, working in the fertile soil, the idea of a Mediterranean diet – its principles and proportions – has always existed, full of flavor and color, and youthfulness. But the passing of time and change to urban living have distracted most of us from the healthy cuisine of our ancestors. Just the same, the populations sur- rounding the Mediterranean Sea continue to maintain dietary habits and lifestyles superior to those of other parts of the world. Perhaps it is the diet, the climate, or the way of life that is responsible or perhaps it is a combination of all these. One thing is certain, the Mediterranean diet is frugal. The term stems from the word "Fruges" which the ancient

XII   THE WAY THEY ATE

Romans used in reference to products of the earth. Everything directs us back to the earth, to the products that come from the soil, and the concept that a frugal diet is necessary to establish and maintain a high level of well-being.

Many individuals deserve to be recognized for this book: professor D'Onofrio, as always, a master; Guido Gnocchi, for his friendship and endless editorial dedication; Gabriella Di Natale, for her enthusiasm and character; Ancel Keys, who, at nearly 100, taught me much about writing; Gabriele Vallefuoco, an excellent technician with images; and all the friends and colleagues with whom I have discussed this project, as well as the authors that have written on this subject; and, finally, my family, for the time that I subtracted from them during the preparation of this work.

Naples, Italy, September 2001   DARIO GIUGLIANO

*To all those in the past
who utilized the Mediterranean
diet without any knowledge
of its benefits*

1 The Mediterranean

The Mediterranean habitat

Long very hot and dry summers, mild and damp winters: these conditions characterize the so-called "Mediterranean climate". Found throughout the world, this is the climate of small areas within temperate latitudes (between the 30th and 40th parallel) where continental land masses face western coasts. The North American Mediterranean is California, in South America it is Chile, in Africa it is Cape Town province, even Australia has two of these areas.

The greater Mediterranean region, which lent its name to this climate, was once known as *Mare Nostrum*. This includes most of southern Europe and the northern coastline of Africa. The Mediterranean is an inland sea, land-locked between continents. The sea is small and its waters are relatively calm. You can sail from coast-to-coast, and when passing through wide-open seas with threatening waves, there is always an island to offer refuge, until better weather comes. The privilege of these conditions has made the Mediterranean a unique focal point on the crossroads of civilization. Its geographic position has assured a great number of human contacts, a variety of relationships and florid trade and cultural exchange. Other even older civilizations, such as the Chinese, advanced alone, but not the Mediterranean. It was continually renewed and enriched by the blending of different cultures. Each marked the prodigious growth of Western civilization which dominated humankind for two millennia.

Around the Mediterranean Sea, plants have adapted to surviving in an environment with a scarcity of annual rainfall and long summer droughts. Some species have developed deep root systems able to tap the underground aquifer. The bulbous plants and herbs reach the

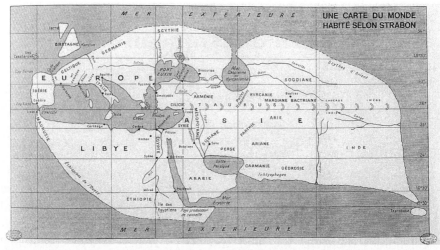

The inhabited world of Strabo. G. Aujac, Strabon, Géographie, livre II, Paris 1969.

height of their growth at the beginning of summer when the soil is still damp; the broadleaf evergreen trees with typical leathery leaves resist drought.

The original Mediterranean landscape was rich and heterogeneous. The high mountains were covered with black pine and cedar. On the gentle slopes, oak faired better at withstanding the heat. Over hill and dale reigned holm oak, and other broadleaf trees. Drought-resistant olive and cork trees colonized the sandstone slopes. At the shoreline, solitary maritime pine often grew skyward with wind-bent trunks.

In classical times the woodland areas of the Mediterranean underwent aggressive deforestation. Plato described the barren and arid hills of the southeastern extremity of central Greece (*Attica*) which had by the 5th century B.C. become denuded.

> *What remains today is like the skeleton of a sick man, because the fertile and soft earth has eroded.*

The many civilizations that flourished in this area caused great changes in the environment. The mountain conifers were cut. Ship builders sought their long and straight trunks. Hardwoods went for charcoal.

The spread of agriculture and
overgrazing led to the destruction
of vast woodland areas in the
foothills. Fortunately, terracing
prevented soil erosion. As time
passed, the ingenious Romans
built a close linked network of
aqueducts and canals to improve
soil irrigation. Crop diversity was
introduced. Olive trees and grapevines were planted on the hills, grain
and other cereals sown on the plains. Exotic plants such as cedar,
pomegranate and fig trees were introduced by merchants and later
farmed on a large scale, even for export. In this fascinating and tor-
mented region of the world, man wrought great havoc, but in the
process learned some innovative farming methods. Hill terracing, irrigation, crop rotation, and fertilizing were practiced since the earliest
recorded history.

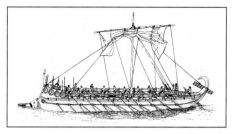

*Model of an Etruscan warship. End of the 6th
century B.C.*

Some species from the original Mediterranean forest have survived,
despite all, and are those that are the most economically important for
farming and grazing in the regions where they grow. The chestnut
forests in Corsica constituted a vital resource and provided flour for

*Small Roman merchant ship loading grain in presence of the tax collector and magistrate.
In the Vatican Museums, Vatican City.*

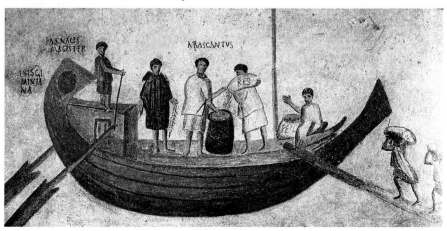

both human and animal consumption. The cork forests of Portugal and Sardinia continue to be commercially important. But the olive remains the most typical Mediterranean tree, the plant that best adapts to the climate of these regions, with its long roots that reach deep for water, its leathery leaves that save moisture and its fruit that swells with oil during the dry season. Like grapevines, fig trees and other plants that have long grown here and may appear to be indigenous, the olive tree is not native to Europe.

The most probable birthplace for the olive tree is Asia Minor and Syria. In these coastal regions, the wild olive tree is, a very common forest tree. Here the Greeks long became aware of this tree, to which they gave the special name λαια. In Latin it was changed to *olea*. Olive tree farming spread by the Greek colonies to the Salentina peninsula, Calabria, Sicily, throughout the Italian peninsula and to the countries around the Mediterranean basin.

The spread of the olive tree to these regions has been influenced by climate and politics, especially as a consequence of various military campaigns or barbarian invasions. From southern Italy the olive tree spread north in the early centuries of the Roman Empire. Large olive groves existed in North Africa during Roman times, were destroyed, and have mostly been replanted. In France the olive tree grew on the banks of the Seine River, then became confined to southern regions. In Spain there was a remarkable expansion in oil production. Even today the nations of the Mediterranean basin still produce more than 90% of all the olive oil in the world.

Grain, oil and wine: the winning triad

The eating habits needed to sustain good health must satisfy the following requirements: supply energy and essential nutritional elements, minimize the risks of chronic disease associated with improper diets and, last but not least, use easily available foods that are safe, tasty and reasonably priced. The diets that best satisfy these criteria are based mostly on fruit, vegetables and cereals. Meat and dairy products play a marginal role in this type of diet.

Throughout history, societies have developed different ways to combine local foods. Traditional ethnic cuisine is the result of this march forward. Studies suggest that traditional cuisines, such as the Mediterranean or Japanese, are associated with a lower incidence of cancer and cardiovascular diseases.

In generic terms, "Mediterranean" refers to a

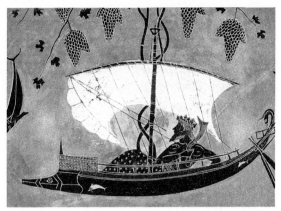

Black-figured cup by Exekias. Dionysus is carried by a sail boat, a grapevine with large bunches of grapes is in the background. Circa 450 B.C. In the Staatliche Antikensammlungen, Munich.

dietary regimen based largely on vegetable products grown and eaten in territories bordering this sea. From one point of view, this term usually identifies the eating habits of the Greeks, southern Italians and other Mediterranean regions where oil represents the main dietary source of fat. This particular type of diet, coupled with an excellent state of health and longevity of the people eating it, is an expression of the common cereal, oil and wine culture passed down directly or indirectly from the ancient peoples living in the Mediterranean basin.

At least 16 countries border the Mediterranean, each with its own cultural heritage, ethnic and religious roots, social and political status, and quite noticeable climatic variations. Of these countries, five are in North Africa, with a rather dry climate, and three are in the Middle East. Some large European countries, such as France, extend beyond the boundaries of the Mediterranean.

Despite the differences influencing individual and collective dietary choices, any society with few special local foods will have them as their common denominator. Although the concept of a Mediterranean diet may appear somewhat artificial for those who barely recall the historical events that have shaped the region over the centuries, the major impact of this culture and the benefits for health have been reported by several authors.

It all begins in Crete

Worried about the need to improve social, economic and sanitary conditions of its people during the post-World War II era, in 1948, the Greek government invited the Rockefeller Foundation to undertake an epidemiological study on the eating habits practiced on the island of Crete. Here was an ethnic group of people with guarded traditions that were centuries old. The goal was to improve the standard of living wherever important nutritional deficiencies emerged. The American team of epidemiologists, lead by Leland Allbaugh, interviewed a random sample of the population. One inhabitant was chosen out of every 150. Information was compiled on several parameters connected with lifestyle. Regarding diet, vegetable foods (cereals, legumes, nuts, potatoes, vegetables and fruit) made up more than 61% of the total daily intake of calories. This was much higher than the 37% reported at that time in the United States.

The surprising thing was that the people of Crete ate the same amount of daily fat as Americans, about 107 grams per day. The remarkable difference was in the quality of fat eaten. Table fats, including oils, comprised 29% of the total energy content for the island inhabitants, versus 15% for the Americans. With the amount of total fats being equal, there was still 14% of energy unaccounted for, that mostly came from saturated animal fats in the American diet. For the islanders, 78% of table fat was from olives and olive oil. The report concluded that the foods eaten in Crete had not undergone any appreciable changes over the centuries: olives, cereals, fruit and vegetables, together with moderate amounts of pork and milk, fish and game. These had remained the staple of the population for 40 centuries.

> ...Everything went with bread...The olives contributed heavily to the energetic intake, so much so that the food appeared to be literally floating in oil...Wine was often drunk, at the main meals...

The eating habits of the people living on Crete in the 50s and 60s led to an excellent state of health. It was better than what would have been expected for a group of people beyond the sphere of Western society and more exposed, they believed, to the harmful effects of poor diet. It was even better than the opulent societies of North Europe and the United States. The model for the Mediterranean diet was born out of these considerations regarding the inhabitants of Crete and spread, almost like wildfire, to embrace the eating habits of other countries producing olive oil.

"Mediterranean diet" is a term ridden with profound symbolic meaning, rendering it unique to this geographical area, the cradle of ancient civilization. The Mediterranean has long been the theater of bloody wars, many of them religious. It has recently been the stage for genocide and racial hatred so unthinkable for people priding themselves on being descendant from so much culture. The Mediterranean basin is the birthplace of the three monotheist religions (Catholic, Islamic, Jewish) that marked the face of history. Could the diet ever unify where politics, religion, and experience have all failed?

What is the Mediterranean diet?

How shall we define what is meant by the Mediterranean diet? For professionals, this term has a precise meaning. This dietary regimen is founded on the eating habits typically found among the inhabitants of the island of Crete, part of continental Greece and South Italy in the early 1960s. The precise temporal and geographic characterization finds its reason for being in the following observations:

– life expectancy in the locations indicated were among the highest in the world despite the poor sanitary conditions. Such a paradox was mostly due to the low incidence of heart disease and some types of cancer;

Black-figured hydria. The main scene represents Tyrrhenian pirates changed into dolphins by Dionysus, narrated in Homer's seventh hymn. 510-500 B.C. In the Museum of Art, Toledo.

- the data relating to the availability of food and to the diet of those peoples permitted researchers to identify common eating habits;
- elsewhere in the world, eating habits based on those common to the Mediterranean basin are linked to a low rate of chronic disease and a long life expectancy.

Once again, therefore, the term Mediterranean diet takes on a well-defined connotation, circumscribed to the Mediterranean basin where the tradition of olive farming is strong.

In the attempt to draw a board outline for this diet, a descriptive summary may be given. Abundant vegetables, fruit, bread, cereals, potatoes, beans, nuts, seeds are the staples. This includes fresh local products such as the fruit eaten at the end of every meal. Overcooked food is discouraged. Sweets made with sugar or honey may be eaten but few times a week. Dairy products (milk, yogurt, cheese) are recommended on a daily basis in limited amounts. Eggs should be limited to 4 per week. Red meat can be eaten in extreme moderation. Wine is drunk at mealtime, with prudence.

A diet of this kind introduces an amount of fat equal to 30% of the total daily energy supply from food. This sometimes fluctuates (25-35%) depending on the region, but it is very low in saturated animal fats, only 7-8% of the total energy supply. The importance of physical activity cannot be stressed enough in the overall relationship between Mediterranean diet and lifestyle.

Regarding that relationship, and considering all the definitions we've mentioned, the Mediterranean diet seems to connote a particularly healthy lifestyle, rather than just a dietary inclination. It is a lifestyle that, in the 1950s, mirrored a series of social and cultural habits of very physically active people. There is a sense of communion one breathes while dining with family or with friends. Lunches are eaten slow to relax and alleviate tension generated by daily stress. The foods are flavorful, well prepared and tastefully presented to stimulate the senses and bolster the concept, even unconsciously, of wholesome diet. And why not take an afternoon nap? Despite its ability to ward off tension, the siesta has gone relatively unappreciated in our age of limitless efficiency. The Mediterranean diet has been deeply rooted in the cultural fabric of the people who benefit from it, without them even knowing it.

The origins

With no written records available, any knowledge of the diet followed by ancient peoples of the Mediterranean basin must come from other sources. The records provided by archaeology help us. Leftover food, especially in tombs, tableware, ceramics, kitchenware, containers to carry provisions, have all been found. What's more, there are numerous clay tablets, papyrus scrolls, parchments and wall etchings that have come to light over many centuries of digs. Finally, literary sources by classical authors, from Homer on, have provided insight. Taken together, these have furnished a picture, with a few gaps, of how ancient peoples ate. They ate a great variety of animal and vegetable products together with bread, spices, sweets, beer and wine.

Written sources, however, that by definition should lend the most credibility, can mislead the reader seeking generalizations on eating habits from only a few references. The Greek heroes described by Homer, for example, ate meat, bread and wine, but paid little attention to vegetables and fruit, perhaps because these were considered vulgar and for the common men. They feared that fresh produce could corrode the dignity of heroes. Olive oil is only cited to glorify its beneficial properties when used as a balm for massages, but always for warriors, never for the common people (*hoi polloi*). With careful reasoning, we can hypothesize that common people, unlike the warriors, always ate vegetables with a heaping of bread and other cereals. In this context, meat and fish, but mostly meat, were eaten only occasionally.

When writing took on more importance, authors began to agree on eating habits. This has been backed by archaeological artifacts describing traditions before the 3rd and 2nd centuries B.C.

We can therefore be reasonably sure that the early written descriptions of the great variety of foods and drinks used and the preparation methods are faithful. Archaeology, art and literature all converge in the knowledge of eating habits of ancient peoples of the Mediterranean. At the same time they furnish indications of the average life expectancy (20-30 years) at the time of Classical Greece and Republican Rome. This short life span was in all likelihood the result of infectious disease and war rather than from famine. Literary sources from that period describe well-nourished citizens. This is a tribute to those civilizations. Be that as it may, less than a century ago, not much had changed: the average life expectancy in Europe at the end of the 19th century was still 40 years.

2 Ancient Egypt

Dining with the Pharaoh

Ancient Egypt left a record of its civilization and everyday life that has come to light thanks to hieroglyphics deciphered by such scholars as Jean-Francois Champollion. These writings have allowed us to reconstruct ever more significant pieces of the splendid mosaic of life in the Nile Valley.

The lives of these people have been safeguarded in painted figures, statues and bas-reliefs. The depictions of triumphant Pharaohs, scenes of people celebrating at feasts and rejoicing through music and dance, body worship through ointments and perfumes, all bear splendid witness to life. Equally suggestive and important to reconstruct history are portrayals of arts and crafts, ceramics craftsmen, farmers, livestock workers, leather craftsmen, stone masons, sculptors, cooks, and barbers. All reveal aspects of the working class and everyday life.

Through the same archaeological sources, portrayals and bas-reliefs have passed down the culinary arts and allowed us to rediscover the foods savored by the ancient Egyptians and their ways of preparing them. Imagine a scene with large feasts and opulent foods for wealthy patrons. This is very different from the frugal diet of the lower class.

There are numerous wall paintings in Egypt of the land along the Nile growing legumes and vegetables (broad beans, lupines, string beans, chickpeas, lentils, squash, cucumbers, onions, garlic, leeks), fruit trees (date and dum-nut, sycamores and pomegranate, fig and peach), barley, spelt, wheat, millet. There are also many scenes of tables sumptuously set with beer, meats and fish, fruit and vegetables. These are the most frequent depictions in tombs to perpetuate scenes of earthly existence.

Vegetables such as onions, garlic, horseradish and cucumbers were an essential part of Egyptian meals. Most people ate them raw. Lettuce was in great demand. Its milky sap was said to make a woman fertile and a man virile. It was endowed with aphrodisiac powers and dedicated to the fertility god Min, who was represented by a phallus symbol wrapped in a tight piece of cloth like a mummy.

Besides being essential, bread was something to take pride in. Great imagination went into producing it in different shapes, and designs, such as buns, or hardtack (eaten by the people living in the desert). Bread was made from wheat or barley. In the New Empire, forty different breads and cakes were made. Of these we know only that they were oval, round or cone-shaped. They looked like fans, vases, and animals, sometimes looking like pyramids, in honor of Imhotep, who built the first stepped pyramid.

Whether rich or poor, every family saw to its own milling and bread making from wheat flour, barley or spelt. Wheat

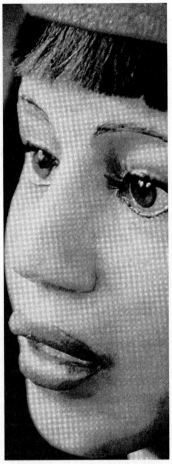

Model of a young Egyptian woman's face.

or barley grains, milled in a stone mortar, were ground on a slanted stone slab. This method allowed them to produce coarse flour. Fine flour was made by roasting and sun drying the grains before grinding. The teeth on most of the Egyptian mummies show signs of ware, likely from mineral dust that formed when flour was made. Dough from flour, salt and water was worked in large containers by feet. The bread was poorly risen or flat. After rising, it was cooked on a stone over the fire or baked in an oven. Even lotus seeds yielded a flour that when mixed with water and milk, made a light digestible bread to be eaten warm. At least this much has been passed down to us by Herodotus:

> When the river is swollen and floods the plain, many lilies, that the Egyptians call lotus, are born from the water. They gather these, dry them in the sun, mill the grain removed from the flower much the same as a corn poppy, and they make bread to bake in the oven. Even the root of the lotus is edible, sweet tasting and is round, as large as an apple.

Tomb paintings and bas-reliefs tell us that the Egyptians favored meat dishes. There are frequent scenes of animal slaughter. This preference for meat was only possible for the wealthy or during sumptuous feasts put on by the Pharaohs. Because of the warm climate, meat preservation was difficult. Meat could be dried to enhance storage. Pigs were raised in large number and their meat played an important role in the regional diet.

More than anything else, the Egyptians ate fowl, from the hunt or from breeding. These mostly included roasted goose and pigeon, but also duck, quail and pelican. The geese and ducks were preserved in large fired clay containers under a layer of fat, perhaps even salt. Roasted goose was portrayed on every decorated table, but even in the most modest tombs, painted limestone models of geese are found ready to be cooked.

Brine pickling and drying geese, duck, quail and other fowl was practiced, as described in ancient times by the Harris Papyrus regarding the preserving of water fowl:

> Open, gutted and dried in the sun.

Goose, pig or beef fat was used to flavor and fry. Oil from sesame seed, linseed, castor-oil, behen-oil from moringa roots, was the most common dressing. Olive oil was known, but its use as a food was limited. Spices, although known, were not used to prepare food, but as medicinal herbs (thyme, cumin).

Fish played a major role in daily diets. However eaten, fresh or sun dried, raw, marinated, salted, roasted or boiled, fish was an important staple for the common people. Numerous species of fish were found in the Nile and in the wetlands of the Delta, in the inland or coastal lakes, in the canals. Other than the species prohibited by religion, all were edible. Herodotus narrated the following phrase:

... and the Egyptians ate great amounts of roasted or boiled fish.

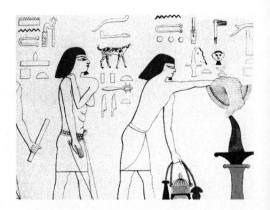

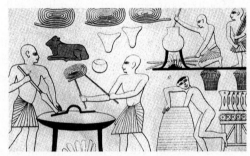

Top. *Kitchenware. Painted by I. Rosellini, Pisa 1834.*

Pastry baking. Monuments of Egypt and Nubia. I. Rosellini, Pisa 1834.

One particular way to preserve fish was to dry it in the sun after having gutted it. It seems that some Babylonian tribes made flour from dried fish by grinding it in a mortar. Such flour was worked into a meal or used to make oven-baked bread. The fondness the Egyptians had for fish can be seen in the portrayals that artistically reveal frames in the lives of fishermen, aspects of fishing and transport ships.

The Egyptians used wild honey from the desert as well as that from bee farming and carob for sweetener. Salt was also commonly used.

The Egyptian diet was rich in legumes (lentils, chickpeas, green peas) and fruit (figs, dates, grapes, sycamore fruit), but also dairy products.

Beer played an absolute pre-eminent role on the Egyptian table. It was commonly used as a drink to toast life. There are many tomb depictions were one can admire such beer drinking scenes.

Wine also contributed to the diet, as well as other more or less alcoholic beverages made from fermenting berries, vegetables or fruit. The
vineyards were well cared for and served to produce table wine. The
first grapevines appeared along the Nile, in the Delta and in the Oases.
The Pharaohs preferred wine from Antylla, near Alexandria. Because of
its steep price, wine was not common among the lower classes, except
during certain festive occasions, perhaps given out by the temple or the
Pharaoh. Wine making was governed by strict rules. Men squeezed the
clusters of grapes with their bare feet in a large tub. The grape juice
was then poured into large amphoras coated on the inside with resin to
seal any leaks and stored away from the sunlight, or buried in the sand
within the cellars. Sometimes the grape juice was cooked and sugared
to make liquor.

Sciedeh was another famous alcoholic drink. This beverage was
made by fermenting wild berries, or fruit. It was drunk mostly by
young men in houses of ill repute. The young were often caught under
the influence of alcohol and reproached for the risks:

> *Do not drink a jar of beer. As you speak, gibberish flows from your
> mouth. If you fall and get hurt, no one will hold your hand to help you
> up. Your friends will stand back and say: to hell with this fool! If some-
> one comes along and asks you questions, you will be on the ground, as
> defenseless as a small child.*

The effects of overdrinking were rapid: in one tomb portrayal an
invited guest of noble standing turns to vomit. Finally, the Insinger
aphorisms have the final word:

> *He who drinks too much wine will be driven to bed by a headache.*

The Egyptian dietary regimen changed the concept of overeating to
wholesome cooking. The following was written by the author of the
Insinger papyrus:

> *Legumes and salt are such fine tasting foods that you can find nothing
> better.*

Many centuries later Herodotus affirmed this about people living on the Nile:

> *The Egyptians use cathartics every month because they believe that foods cause most diseases.*

The common man was thoroughly convinced that good health depended on ones ability to eat his fill: a big eater was in shape, disease-free and in peace with the world.

As for the timetable of meals, it appears that they followed a well cadenced plan. That is to say, breakfast came in the morning, lunch was taken at midday and supper eaten in the evening. Fruit or home-made bread and vegetable snacks were also figured into the day. These meals were all washed down with the most important drink of all – beer. The Egyptians set their tables only with trays of food, while young naked maidens served drinks, but this happened at feasts organized by the well off, on important occasions.

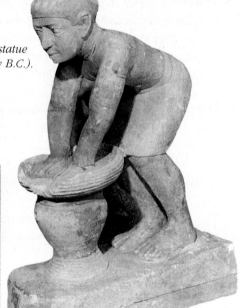

Man making beer. Painted limestone statue from the 5th dynasty (25th-23th century B.C.). In the Museum of Cairo.

A milking scene. A bas-relief from a Kawit sarcophagus. 11th dynasty (2134-1991 B.C.). In the Museum of Cairo.

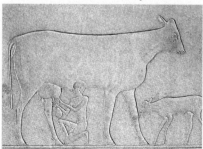

No cookbooks have survived, but the Egyptians are believed to have been good cooks and, above all, liked to eat.

It seems that the Egyptians ate with their hands. This is confirmed by the presence of basins behind or under the tables to rinse hands during the meal, as can be seen in the scene in Horemheb's tomb. At a nobleman's table it was customary to eat alone or with no more than two seated around the table. Feasts were different. They were enlivened by music and dance, with garlands that encircled the wine and beer amphoras, by the scent of lotus buds that the guests with flower crowns exchanged with each other.

Sitting at the table with an ancient Egyptian would not be disappointing. One would have to do without the fruits we usually eat because oranges, lemons and bananas were unknown to him, whereas cherries, almonds, peaches and pears only made their appearance during Roman times. Yet there would be nothing to worry about. For meat lovers, excellent steaks would be there to taste, or filet mignon or flank steaks, all chosen pieces cooked on the grill. And then there would be fish and fowl, every kind of garden vegetable in abundance, eaten with an exquisite fragrant home baked bread. One wouldn't be without dessert, tarts cooked with butter and made more appetizing with cream and honey. One's meal would end with fruit such as dates, figs, apples, watermelon and melons. To drink, teetotalers could choose water or milk. All others could drink highly acclaimed delta wine, while beer, the ever-present national drink of the Egyptians, would be flowing. There would, naturally, be subtle differences from table to table. For example, the Pharaoh's banquet was different from the frugal meal eaten by a farmer or craftsman. The one common ground, judging from remaining records, was the use of fingers instead of forks. Noblemen or commoner, sovereign or proletariat, all Egyptians ate like this.

Eternal life with food

The archeologist was carrying out excavations in a particularly scenic area, where the Saqqarah plain is like a desert spur jutting into the grassland that stains the feet of anyone who walks through it. The royal

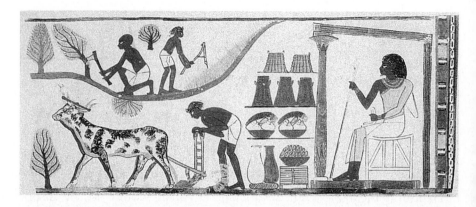

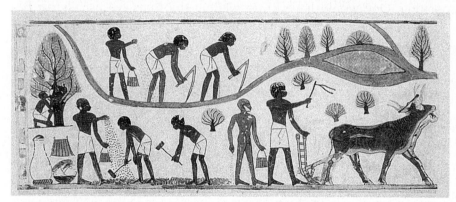

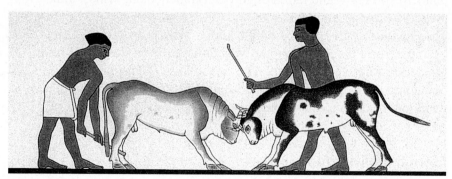

Scenes of farming and rearing livestock. The administrator Nakht overseeing tillage and seeding (upper panels). Tomb of Nakht at Thebes. Herdsmen stop two bulls from fighting (painting by Prisse d'Avennes).

tomb of Pharaoh Zoser, the famous stepped pyramid, was a still silhou-
ette in the desert. Tradition has it that Imhotep, the most famed physician in all of ancient Egypt, who the Greeks renamed Asclepios god of
medicine, had it built for the Pharaoh's glory. In taking that shape the
pyramid suggested a change in the relationship between sovereign and
subjects. From a simple *mastaba*, funeral room dug out of the rock, the
stepped pyramid grew by overlapping parallelepiped gradations. The
ruling class view of reality, depicted in the tombs, became by simple
translation the way the people thought.

The moment's excitement had infected the group of excavators. A
group of archaic tombs had already come to light. The largest was extraordinary, not so much for the size of the central mound, as for the
wall around it, which was rectangular and enclosed the massive structure that carried the same number of rows of individual tombs on three
sides. The bodies of the individuals preserved in these tombs must
have belonged to domestics and house servants that the owner of the
tomb brought with him into the designed for the hereafter. But the
choice must have been voluntary, troublesome, yet without any forcing. It implys such an important advantage in accepting the high cost of
death. This advantage was a prerogative not allowed to all. It was a
guarantee of life continuous with the master in his eternal home, in a
world beyond, where the functions and activities carried out before
death would remain unchanged.

The emerging edifice at ground level had a series of rooms for use,
as in a true house; storage rooms to accumulate enormous numbers of
vases containing dining ware (1500 stone and 3500 terracotta vases),
and the supplies for the hereafter. In one undefiled room, alabaster, terracotta or diorite plates brimming with food were found beside the sarcophagus of a woman. All of these wares were perfectly recognizable
after fifty centuries. There was a baby's barley cereal, a cooked quail,
two kidneys perhaps from sheep, a headless fish, eight prime ribs of
beef, small round cakes, cooked figs, grapes, large jars with wine and
beer, and small vases containing cheese.

The discovery of this tomb belonging to a remote lady from the 2nd
dynasty (2700 B.C.) brought the tomb of the architect Kha, from a
much earlier period (1400 B.C.), to the archaeologist's recollection. That

burial site was also found intact and rich in furnishings and ample supplies such as bread, flour packed into a vase, grain, cheese, cuts of meat and fowl, dried fish, and salt in a wooden container. Vases also contained algae, onions, and much fruit, grapes, dates, juniper berries and cumin seeds, a posthumous witness to a varied and balanced diet.

The deceased individual from that tomb is depicted as a table companion. He sits at the table lavished with all kinds of food, an obsessive repetition that fit the belief of continued life after death, trusted to the care of the living that saw to the depositing of food and drink.

The Egyptians were not willing to accept the end of life. Death was a passage; a different stage of life. They believed that man could save his own identity after death. This sentimental willingness not to see the necessary end in death, was the foundation of the importance attributed to a series of ceremonies performed on the mummified body and anteceding the offerings of food, drink, clothing and perfumes.

The first and indispensable condition to assure a happy stay in the hereafter for the deceased was the preservation of the body. For the Egyptians, the body did not represent an ephemeral home for the spirit to leave only momentarily to met the god Ra in the underworld. If the body were to decompose, the soul would not be able to return and would be lost forever. In the second book of *Histories*, Herodotus narrates that, after funeral rites, the body was brought to the funeral home to be embalmed. This procedure lasted about 30 days, even 70 days if the deceased was a dignitary, a king, a queen or a Pharaoh. Thus, an inscription in the tomb of a high ranking official of the Pharaoh Tuthmosis III:

> *You will certainly have a beautiful funeral, after which the 70 days of your embalming will take place, you will be placed upon a coffin and be pulled by white bulls... A funeral sacrifice will be offered to you.*

The poor had to satisfy themselves with a quick and low cost embalming; everyone had to guard themselves against vile profanation that, rumor had it, occurred in the funeral homes when the deceased was a beautiful and esteemed woman. In that case, the cadaver was delivered three or four days old and in an advanced state of decomposition to impede the embalmers from taking carnal liberty.

The Egyptian aware that even a mummified cadaver ran the risk of destruction came to the novel idea of survival without cadaver preservation. One or more statues representing the defunct were placed in the tomb so that the soul could be preserved should the body deteriorate, or even spare heads, while the name of the expired person was carved several times into the walls of the tomb and on the objects contained within. Even the name could assist the deceased. As a last measure of security, small statues called *ushebti* were sealed within the tomb. Their job was to serve the dead in the hereafter, and substitute for him should he be called to work.

Looking at the canopic vases, the archeologist pondered the meaning of Papyrus Rhind I, where the four Canopic Vessels, the genies that protected the viscera of the dead, gave testimony to the enjoyable and material existence that the deceased had arranged for his body.

> *He did not mistreat us during his life! We drank every day until drunkenness, we ate goose and fish to our heart's content... we drank the good stuff, we slept well, we always had food befitting of humans placed before us, and that is how we aged on the earth.*

Along the Nile

Egypt has long been considered a gift of the Nile. Many centuries before Herodotus, while forging the river, a man named Hanis admired the usual landscape that evoked in him ever-new emotions and thought about the importance of water. Like everyone else, Hanis was aware that if the river had not had its particular rhythm, agriculture would only have been possible in the fields along its banks. But his sight rested upon the fields, vegetable gardens and fruit groves; not a single square centimeter of ground went uncultivated, claimed by wood, lawn, or simple shrubland.

That year, in August, the river waters overflowed their banks with the usual ferocity, covering the inland valley for many kilometers. Now, with the arrival of autumn, the waters were receding and moist silt covered the land, making it ready for planting.

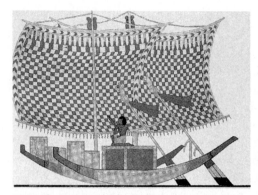

Painting by Ippolito Rosellini (Pisa 1834) depicting an Egyptian ship.

The plain, however, did not always take on a beneficial appearance. Last year and the one before that, the fast and violent flow of water had risked causing a catastrophe: fortunately, the drainage ditches softened the rush and local populations were able to use it to their advantage. All things considered, human labor seemed to bring out the true miracle of the Nile.

Hanis' boat moved against the flow, but with only four oarsmen at his disposal, that task did not come easy. The beat of the mallet kept a steady rhythm for the rowers. They panted from the work and the heat.

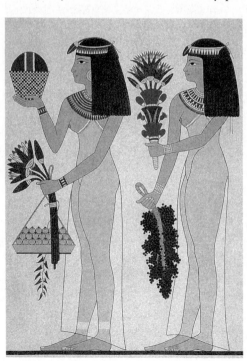

Traffic on the river was heavy at that hour of the day. There were overloaded straw rafts with stone blocks, fishermen, and people lingering on boats anchored away from shore. One large vessel slid swiftly upstream powered by eight rowers. It was a deluxe craft with dignitaries, perhaps visiting their farms. The flooding was over and the waters were

Oblations made by young women in ceremonial dress: transparent linen tunics with crossing shoulder straps, wide collars, diadems and garlands in their hair. They carry figs, bunches of grapes, flowers and basket of food. Histoire de l'Art Egyptien, Prisse d'Avennes, 1858-1877.

returning to the riverbed. In a short while seeds were to be sown: usually, wheat, sorghum, flax and barley were rotated.

Seated on the clean smelling straw, Hanis happily savored the dishes brought to him by a slave girl: brined fish, mutton browned over scented coals, snail-shaped bread, dried fruit and beer. Oh! The beer, what a delicious drink. But you had to put your heart into making it; otherwise the acid taste that it acquired would ruin the drink. Having worked for a certain time in the sector, Hanis well remembered the various steps to prepare beer. In his mind's eye he saw the women grinding barley, mixing it with water, and envisioned the forms baking in the oven. An energetic stirring started the fermentation process. Finally, the filtrated slurry was ready to drink. They made dark beer (*bag*) or light lager (*send*). Those who produced large quantities, such as the farms that made it, could sell it to Egyptian or foreign merchants.

From time to time boats loaded with hay and stores of food, papyrus plants and amphoras of oil glided alongside his craft, in the opposite direction, leaving a white wake that reflected the crimson rays of the setting sun. Whenever this occurred it caused his heart to throb. From the warmth of his heart sprang the memory of Kati and her beautiful house. Kati's home was on the banks of the Nile, immersed in luxuriant foliage. The gardens were planted with legumes and vegetables (mostly broad beans and string beans), but also lettuce, squash and surrounding it were fruit trees (palms and dates, sycamores and pomegranates). Near the shore, cane thickets and marshes bloomed with vegetation. There were green papyrus and lotus (the symbol of eternal life), water nymph, bed of rushes and uncountable herbs and wetland plants. The vast garden was lost among the acacia, the yew, the tamarind and the cuckoo plants. An artistic arbor stood beneath three large sycamores where supper was taken on summer evenings.

He remembered all the meals he had eaten there while sitting on low walls or small tables:

> *The servants set before them several kinds of beer, and different focaccia breads, helpings of vegetables, and every species of fruit for refreshment.*

Hanis thoroughly enjoyed the pastries shaped like animals, made from wheat flour mixed with honey and dried grapes. Kati had a weakness for those shaped like dolls that children are so fond of, kneaded with dates or carob. Not even the sight of the other cakes made with flour dough rolled to a spiral, and then fried in large pans filled with oil could dissuade her. To the east were the kitchens, the servant's quarters, the courtyard with silos, the stores of grain and food supplies.

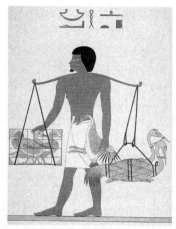

It would have been a fine life if only the greedy scribes would not torment the peasant farmers with so many taxes, forcing them to pay revenue on the bases of a presumed harvest, even before seeding. Little did they care if excessive drought or adverse weather conditions caused the earth to render up little. Taxes were to be paid,

A servant carrying ducks and cranes (drawing by Prisse d'Avennes).

or there would be harsh punishment such as strong beatings or mutilation. This state of affairs had a negative impact; above all, it failed to guarantee the domestic tranquility so coveted by the Pharaoh.

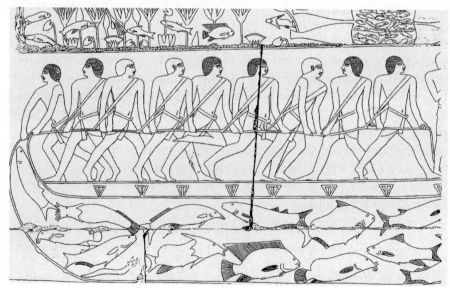

Fishing with a net. Tomb of Mereruke. 6th dynasty (second half of the 3rd millennium B.C.).

Fishing in the land of the papyrus

In one Egyptian writing dating to the 12nd dynasty (twenty centuries before Christ), the so-called *Satire of Trades* regarding fishermen, someone named Kheti instructed his son Pepi:

> *Let me tell you something about a fisherman. He suffers more than anyone else does, because his job is on the river, in the midst of crocodiles.*

The importance of fishing for the ancient Egyptians is evident from the number of times it occurs in scenes decorating the tombs of private citizens, or Sovereign, for whom fishing was a favorite pastime. In a manuscript from the 12nd dynasty, a fishing trip to the Fayum cane thickets was organized by courtesans who were worried about the overworked Sovereign. Today, this place is still known for the fine quality of its fish.

One fishing scene is depicted in Nebwenef's tomb. The Theban high priest is pictured fishing with a reed pole on the banks of a canal while sitting on a throne. A butterfly resting on the pole indicates serenity. Such images reinforce the concept that fishing was considered a pleasant and relaxing pastime.

Salt water fishing, and even more importantly, river fishing in the Nile played an important role in the country's diet and economy. Herodotus makes the following remark:

> *When the river waters recede, fish deposit their eggs in the last puddle of water remaining. These hatch with the next flooding. For this reason the Nile is never without fish.*

The fishing techniques of the ancient Egyptians were not unlike those used today. They used nets and hooks, with or without rods. Certainly fishing with a net reaped better yields. Funeral depictions describe this following scene: alongside each other with a taut net between them, two crews made a semicircle holding one end of the net, or simply drawing a net full of fish up on dry land. Fishing in shallow water was more rewarding when performed with fish traps or wicker baskets.

Despite organized fishing, the practice was regulated by rather strict laws. It appears that priests were granted the right to fish, and bestowed this onto fishermen. This can be read in the papyrus from Fayum. Again from the papyrus we learn that fishermen had a substantial income, and that they were placed under surveillance as a result. They could not, for example, catch some species such as *lepidotus* and eels because they were held to be sacred. Even *oxyrynchus*, the fish said to have swallowed Osiris' private parts, could not be eaten in some areas of the country. Relating to this, in one writing fourteen fishmongers from Fayum boasted that they had never been branded with the accuse of catching such fish nor eating them. Among the sacred fish was the *tilapia*. When associated with the flooding of the Nile, it came to symbolize renewed life and fertility. When associated with lotus flowers (symbol of regeneration), it became a cherished decorative element on painted bowls.

With the exception of some species, fish was an important food for the ancient Egyptians, but was prohibited for priests. Its use was so widespread and common that it was not held to be a worthy meal for the deceased or Sovereign. For religious purposes the Egyptians mummified some kinds of fish and buried them in specially constructed necropolises to symbolize hope of resurrection to new life. In Khabethnet's tomb in Thebes (19th dynasty, 1293-1185 B.C.) there is in fact a portrayal of the god Anubis embalming a huge fish, projection of the desire for resurrection.

Herodotus mentioned that the Egyptians ate roasted or boiled fish. Egyptians living in the swamps even ate it raw after gutting and drying it in the sun. This way of preserving fish, foreseeing the periods of shortage, has been passed down over the millennia. Still today, there are places in Africa where children are given the chore of guarding fish that have been cleaned and dried in the sun.

Archaeological descriptions and icons reveal that the most prized fish was the *lates* both for the taste of its meat and for its eggs. These were eaten fresh of dried. Two species of mullet that date to the first floodgates still live in the Nile. Their eggs are called *batarakh* and are still a delicacy in Egyptian cuisine. Still, there are no traces of the recipes used in daily fish preparation, nor those for ancient feasts.

3 The daring Phoenicians

At the Phoenician table

The Phoenician nation formed a strip of land between the mountain chain of Lebanon, the AntiLebanon range, and the sea. What little farmland the Phoenicians had was fertile. The true Phoenician civilization set its roots into the broad cultural base of the near East. It is likely that these near-eastern traditions persisted even for nutrition. Syrian, Assyrian, Egyptian, Israeli and Greek literature give us an inkling of culinary arts in this region.

Phoenician meals were laden with farm products, wheat and barley. The Bible tells us of cereal in Phoenicia and in the nearby geographic areas. Barley and wheat were the trading goods between Israel and the Phoenician city of Tyros during Solomon's reign. Egypt, too, was indicated by the prophet Isaiah as a rich supplier of wheat. These recorded histories suggest Phoenicia's inability to meet production demands for the size of the population through extensive farming – despite the fertility of their land – because of the limited available space.

Cereals were eaten boiled – consumed this way throughout the near East since prehistoric times – or made into bread, including different types of *focaccia* breads. The cooking methods for cereal used by the Phoenicians have largely been deduced from other sources. The Bible, at least in reference to ritual offerings, mentions two different types of utensils used: a *focaccia* bread pan and a type of frying or starchy food pan. At the temple of Astarte, at Kition, the Phoenician colony on Cyprus, *focaccia* breads prepared by staff bakers at the temple were offered. In particular, one inscription mentions the offering of *focaccia* breads made with juniper berries.

In the region of ancient Syria-Palestine, cereal or various parts of plants (pods, seeds, leaves) were blended with legumes into flour. This

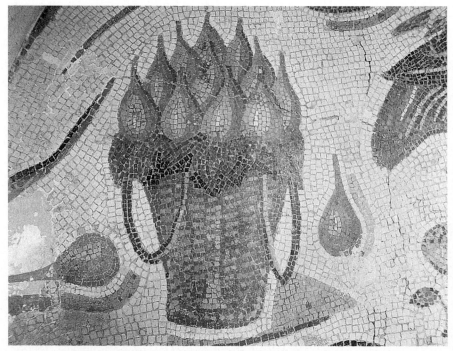

Mosaic of a basket filled with figs. 4th century B.C. In the Museum of Bardo, Tunis.

is clear from economic records from Ugarit as well as the Bible. In his writings, Pliny the Elder provided a description of a treatment for wheat and barley, which is still used by north African villages. Wheat and barley were the prime grains in ancient societies where bread and oil were the staples and mythological symbols of existence.

As for bread, the yeast-risen variety coexisted with long lasting ship's biscuits, so essential for a nation of sailors. Using common recipes, different flours were made into mush, semolina and similar dishes.

Placed high on the list of food rations in Ugarit were lentils. The story of how Esau traded his birthright for a bowl of lentils is well known, while the second book of Samuel cites how a warrior defends a field of lentils from the Philistines (a Sea People).

Garlic, onions, leeks, cucumbers had to have been known in the region – Pliny tells us of them in his *Naturalis Historia* – and from

Ascalon, the Philistine city, we get the name scallion (*allium ascalinicum*). Squash has been reported in use since Hellenistic times. As for garlic, it seems that the Phoenicians used it extensively in their cooking.

Hors-d'oeuvres were in accepted use in Phoenician cuisine, as were various tidbits and appetizers, cooked in grape leaves (as in Greece and Calabria, Italy) and the authentic crepes-Suzette, double layers of dough with honey filling.

The embroidered and jagged coastline was easily fished for crab, lobster, and shellfish, mullet, gilthead, sea bass and tuna, to end up with *garum*, the most celebrated and notorious fish sauce ever made. This was prepared from the insides of tuna, sturgeon, mackerel and the cannibal morays. Much has been recorded about this sauce, which has become a Mediterranean legend, albeit mostly derogatory. This does not subtract from the fact that for centuries it was the rage of these shores. In a malicious pun, writer Martial refers to an unfortunate gentleman by the name of Papilus who changes a delicate fragrant flower into *garum* just by breathing on it.

Salt mining went hand in hand with the fish industry. Information passed down from *Ugaritic palatin* manuscripts mention it as the only seasoning. It is likely that salt then spread to Phoenician cities.

Those who were well off chose to eat wild game or livestock. Particular rituals were derived from animals drawn from herds of cattle and sheep. The climate did not lend itself to preserving or drying such meat. Barnyard animals were often eaten; chickens, rabbits, pigeons, and more rarely, pigs and cattle. Poultry was the most widely used food in Carthaginian meals. It appears that the rearing of livestock began with the Phoenicians. Certainly wild game must have played only a marginal role in providing meat. The Bible mentions it only rarely and the Egyptian Sinuhe, in his imaginative account speaks of it as a highly considered food, destined for a well-to-do table.

Milk and dairy products together with honey, the universal sweetener, played an important role. Bee farming reigned in the land of Assyria-Babilonia. In the Bible, Canaan of the Phoenicians is running over with honey. In fact, the Biblical definition of Canaan is the "land of milk and honey". Beyond all the literary and allegoric interpretations given, this certainly indicates how highly they considered the white beverage. Its production and use were tied to breeding that must have been thriving. Milk was one of the products that Tyros, meaning in a broad sense the entire region, imported from Judea and Israel, and must have even been used to make cakes.

Cheese is cited in a Ugaritic manuscript dealing with the dairy industry. The Old Testament repeatedly mentions butter and sour milk. Thus, it may be assumed that these dairy products were also used in Phoenician territory. Was it not a coincidence that Jael served it to the Cananite Sisara before putting him to death?

The Phoenicians were guaranteed proteins and carbohydrates, fats and mineral salts in their ancient diet. They had no relative vitamin deficiencies common elsewhere. Thus, their alert minds, brisk bodies and keen senses were never dampened.

Fruit tree farming was widespread. Dates, figs, apples, pomegranates and quince apples, almonds, pistachios, citron and persimmons were mentioned in Assyrian and Babylonian texts, in the Bible and, later, in writings by classical authors.

The Bible mentions figs some fifty times, almost to affirm its use throughout Palestine, and the Phoenician fig was still renown in Egypt during Hellenistic times. It is worth noting that fresh or dried figs are so sweet that they could substitute for more expensive sweeteners, such as honey, which was surely destined for the rich and regal tables. Dates were still imported into Athens from Phoenicia in the 5th century B.C.

As a flavoring, this ancient ingenious people used olive oil. It was almost a consequential dessert for Phoenician and then Punic feasts and very much part of the classical Mediterranean diet. Oil was made from olives and from other oil producing seeds. It was indispensable as a source of lipids in the daily diet. It seems to have been reported for the first time in the 2nd millennium in Syria and in Palestine. In Ugarit the remains of oil producing sites along with numerous pieces of large containers designed to hold the precious liquid have been located in early bronze age strata. Oil farming started in Phoenicia.

Some administrative documents from Ugarit (where grape presses already existed in the 3rd millennium) dating to the 14th-13th century B.C., mention large terraced vineyards that guaranteed a copious supply of wine for royal warehouses. Moreover, names were given to the clay pots used to store and use wine. There were large jars to save wine and chalices to drink it in. Except for the wine named *passum*, it seems that Phoenician wines were not of great taste. A particular Lebanese wine is recurrent in biblical exaltation and also remembered by its perfumed fragrance of incense by Pliny the Elder. Was this perhaps *retsina*, an early version of Greek resined wine? It is thus not hard to imagine that the ancient Phoenicians delighted in succulent fig wine, just as we know that they were gluttons of *passum* made with very sweet dried grapes and without doubt the precursor of our analogous dessert wines.

Beer and other drinks made by fermenting cereals were not widely used. Another beverage mentioned by Pliny the Elder and used in the region of Utica was herb tea made mostly from husked barley.

Dining in Carthage

The people of Carthage were masters of good cooking. Punic recipes were in vogue throughout the Greek and Roman world. Plautus, and all others living in the Mediterranean basin, described the Carthaginians as soup eaters (*Pultiphagonides*).

Carthaginian land was fruitful. Wheat and barley abounded. As a result, the Carthaginians had several first courses. The best known of all, especially for its high nutritional value, was Punic soup. This was called *puls punica* by Plautus. The meal was a true precursor of a single course. It was nutritious with all of the carbohydrates, fats, proteins and to a lesser extent, vitamins, provided by the cereals, cheese, honey and eggs. We even have Cato's recipe:

> *Put a pound of flour into water and mix well, pour it into a clean tub and add three pounds of fresh cheese, half a pound of honey and one egg, mix well and cook in a new pot.*

Raised bread and hard tack were in wide use. The Romans knew of the fragrant *punicum*, a pleasant *focaccia* bread made with cereal flours. Still today, bread and *focaccia* breads are cooked in small terra-cotta ovens wherever Africa is bathed by the Mediterranean. Wheat was so important that it was stamped onto Carthaginian coins and on those of its Sardinian colonies.

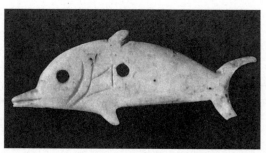

As for legumes, Cato cites the Punic chickpea and Pliny the Elder proposes a method to mash lentils, taken from a text written by Mago, known Carthaginian agronomist from the 4th century B.C. His work has in part been passed down by Roman authors.

Punic ivory carving of a dolphin. 5th-3rd century B.C. In the National Archeology Museum of Cagliari, Sardinia.

First toast the lentils, then mash them lightly with bran...

Classical sources describe luxurious vegetable gardens in Carthage and speak of cabbage, and the highly prized cardoon, grown for the affluent tables, as well as artichokes and garlic. Pliny the Elder defines Cyprus *ulpicum* as a very famous rustic food.

The fishing industry was one of the most florid for the economy. Gades, the current Cadiz, was known to classical authors for its fish salting plants and for the production of *garum*. Besides eating shellfish and lobster, revealed by archaeological digs, they ate gilthead, mullet, sturgeon, moray, sea bass and tuna.

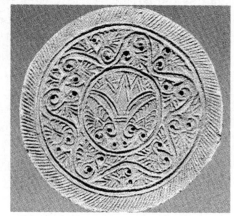

Milk and dairy products were provided by farm animals (horses and cattle), that were, in particular circumstances, slaughtered for meat. The Carthaginians disdained pork, but did not abhor dog meat. Barnyard animals, such as chicken, rabbit and pigeon were eaten regularly.

Clay seal for focaccia bread. 6th-5th century B.C. In the National Archeology Museum of Cagliari, Sardinia.

The remains of eggshells in tombs testify to their use and show the importance that eggs had in making *puls punica*. Eating ostrich eggs must have been rare and limited to the areas bordering on that animal's habitat.

Carthaginian honey from bee farming was particularly appreciated along with the quality wax derived from this source.

Side dishes of fruit and vegetables enhanced the Carthaginian menu, particularly at wealthy tables. They ate cardoon, artichokes, cabbage, chickpeas, pomegranate, almonds, nuts, pears, dates and figs. Pliny the Elder again cites different species of pears and apples and defines pomegranate as *malum punicum*, praising the quality and quantity of Carthaginian production. We have Mago's recipe to save the freshness of pomegranates:

> *Wrap the freshly picked apples [pomegranates] with a layer of well mixed potter's earth; when this clay dries, hang it in a cool place; before eating, put it in water to devolve the earth.*

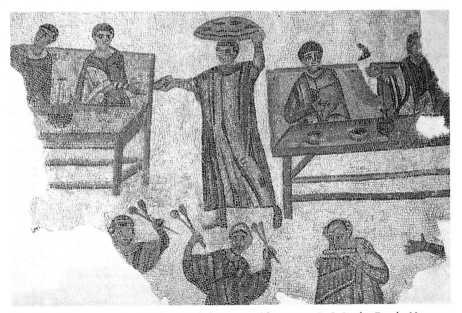

Mosaic with a scene of a Carthaginian banquet. 4th century B.C. In the Bardo Museum, Tunis.

Carthaginian figs were so good, and had such wide fame that they were exported to Greece and Rome. Standing before the Roman people, Cato demonstrated just how close the threat of Carthage was by revealing a fig he had picked in that city. Shells from walnuts, hazelnuts and almonds have been found in some tombs in Carthage and in Sicily (Lilibeo). They ate pistachio nuts, chestnuts and many dates; grapes were eaten fresh or dried in the sun.

There was a law in Carthage that regulated wine consumption. According to Pliny the Elder, the quality of Carthaginian wine was not very good because lime was added as a sweetener. It is likely that the dissemination of wine as a beverage occurred at a later date, perhaps towards the end of the 5th century B.C., when written sources attribute wine importation from other Mediterranean countries.

Columella gives us Mago's recipe for *passum*, the famous wine made from raisins:

> *Pick the first bunches when very ripe, throw away the rotten or moldy grapes...hang the bunches high up on reeds exposed to sunlight, cover at night to avoid dampness; once dried, pick the grapes from the bunches and throw them into a jar or into a jug; pour in grape must, the best possible, until the grapes get covered. On the sixth day, put it all into a tub and squeeze it with a wine screw press and save the juice; then press the raw wine, adding fresh wine must made from other grapes left in the sun for three days; mix well and put it through the wine press. Seal this second pressed wine immediately in airtight clay pots...; then, after twenty or thirty days, when fermentation stops, pour it into other pots; immediately whitewash the covers with plaster and cover it all with a skin.*

Again Mago, in his book on agriculture written at the time of the Punic wars, furnishes precious advice for grape farming:

> *Train the runners north, to reduce damage from heat; place stones in the holes to be planted, to guard against winter flooding; introduce raw wine mixed with manure, to favor root growth; do not fill in the hole right away, but do it little by little, to push the roots deep.*

Carthage produced oil. The most famous olive trees were the *miliarii*. The name comes again from Pliny and refers to the annual weight of oil, almost 327 kilograms. It seems that olive tree farming was brought by the Phoenicians to Carthage in North Africa. Pliny gives us an idea of what olive farming was like:

> *In the shade of the superb palm, grow olive trees, beneath the olives, grow the fig trees; below the figs, grow the pomegranate trees, under them the grapevines; under the vines, grow wheat, then legumes, finally, salad greens: all in the same year and all the plants get nourished in the shade of the other.*

The region around Carthage was fertile, rich with vineyards, olive groves, fruit trees and pastureland. Inland, the highly taxed Libyans farmed the land that produced grain in abundance to meet the needs of the city. The reporters after Agathocles, who were the first to bring Roman teachings to Africa, were fascinated by the fertility of the soil and production of the land.

The Carthaginians were master bakers. They made flour pastries, and above all, as the Roman Festus Avienus described, a cake called *pobum* (delicious) for whose possession the gluttonous Romans had even justified the Punic wars.

Black ships

The Phoenicians were bold explorers. They were the first to challenge the oceans and circumnavigate Africa. Sailors and pirates, on their black ships guided by the small bear constellation, touched the mythical land of Ofir and grazed Thule. They invented fast ships, were shrewd and had a sense of direction. They explored both land and sea. They crossed the deserts by caravan, and the seas by vessel. Everywhere they went they opened markets and built ports. The black ships berthed at every port in the Mediterranean. The men came ashore wearing long tunics without belts, rings hung from their ears. They were followed by a procession of slaves laden with bales of wares to set up on the beach.

Then they climbed back aboard their ships and sent up smoke. The local inhabitants seeing the smoke neared the shore, they piled gold in exchange next to the goods and retreated. The Carthaginians went ashore again: if they judged the quantity of gold worthy, they took it and left, otherwise they returned to their ships.

This scene comes from Herodotus, who wrote the words five hundred years before Christ. But it calls to mind even older scenes, repeated for thousands of years.

The Phoenicians were therefore merchants, but most of all, they were great explorers. As their population grew, however, food stores became scarce. To get wheat, wine and oil from other nations more blessed by nature, they turned to the sea, to trading. They became very skilled craftsmen, and their wares were goods to be traded. They thus

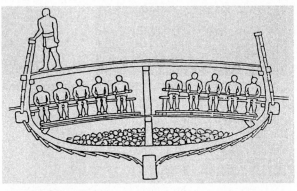

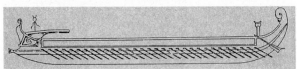

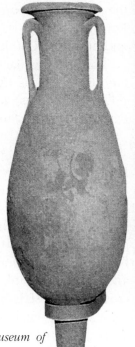

Top. *Reconstructed transverse section of the forward part of a Carthaginian ship. 3rd century B.C.*

Drawing of a Carthaginian ship. 3rd century B.C.

Right. *Amphora for garum. 1st-2nd century B.C. In the Museum of Carthage, Tunisia.*

became great navigators. The Phoenicians were therefore not colonizers, they did not transplant their surplus population like the Greeks. They were anxious to establish sea links, port calls and markets, to set up a close commercial network. Everywhere they stopped to unload goods and load others, the ships left merchants ashore. They made quick deals. These were the forerunners of door-to-door salesmen, who went about from village to village to sell Phoenician craftsmanship, such as pottery, metal goods and jewelry. Upon their return, they were loaded with what they received in trade. They had large amounts of wheat, amphoras of oil, or roles of cloth, pieces of gold or silver, even slaves.

The Phoenicians sought above all metals, cereals, exotic and precious materials along the Mediterranean routes. They did not scorn the slave trade, the fruit of some raid. The description of a Phoenician in Homer's Odyssey is particularly interesting:

An expert in trickery, a thief who left very bad deeds among men.

And again:

Famous navigators, but rascals, who carry endless knick-knacks on their black ships (rubbed with pitch).

Their trade expansion into the Mediterranean basin began in the 12th century B.C., in the wake of political and economic turmoil that followed the destructive surge of the Sea Peoples. By about 1100 B.C. they were in Tunisia and on the Atlantic coast of Spain; in the 9th century there is news of Phoenician settlement on Cyprus, Malta and Sardinia. A century later they were in Sicily. But already since the start of the 9th century, merchants from Tyros had established the berth at Carthage, the new city, would be named the lady of that sea. By importing massive quantities of grain from Sardinia and silver from Spain, Carthage became the richest city in the world, but its dominion was based upon the economic oppression of subjected peoples who nourished only hatred towards those who lived by extortion. Carthage long contested the dominion of the sea with the Sicilian Greeks and fatally ended up colliding with the growing Roman expansion. In the mortal conflict that lasted more than a century (264-164 B.C.), Rome held the upper hand and destroyed its hated rival.

Around 425 B.C. a heavily manned Carthaginian fleet under the command of Annone rounded the straits of Gibraltar and gave start to one of the boldest feats in ancient times: the exploration of Africa's Atlantic coast. This mythical adventure lasted years and brought awareness of an area hitherto unknown called "desert country." The log of that mission, compiled by Annone, was posted at the temple of Baal Hammon in Carthage, although the document handed down to us is a Greek translation that had been safeguarded in Delphi, city of the oracle and collection center for all information regarding Mediterranean peoples. The journey ended in Sierra Leone, or more likely, Cameroon and Gabon. Again, the search for precious metals drove the Phoenicians to daring feats:

> *We heard the sounds of flutes and cymbals, the rumble of drums and loud screams. With that we were gripped with fear and the soothsayers ordered us to abandon the island. Quickly distancing ourselves [from there], we passed nearby a scorching place, rich with exotic smells, where swelling hot streams rushed to the sea. We could not stay because of the heat. Therefore, terror-stricken, we moved away from there.*

In written history, the Phoenician navigators came upon the scene with the annals of Pharaoh Tuthmosis III (1500 B.C.) who embarked his troops in the Nile Delta on Cananite ships. Cananite, at least in the Old Testament, was another name used to designate the Phoenicians.

Although the oldest glass objects found so far come from Egypt, about 2500 years before Christ, and then from Babylon, almost in the same period, and from Ediru, a Sumerian city (2200 B.C.), classical tradition attributes the Phoenicians with the invention of glass. The invention was a lucky combination of silicon dioxide with sodium, potassium, calcium or magnesium. Pliny the Elder describes it in his *Naturalis Historia*:

> *The story is that a ship with saltpeter merchants once set ashore at a certain place and strewed themselves on the beach to prepare lunch. Since*

it happened that no stones of adequate size were available to maintain the pot, they brought pieces of saltpeter down from the ship. When these heated up and mixed with the beach sand a new type of transparent liquid began to gush. This, it is said, is the origin of glass.

The Phoenicians were not only ship builders, but glass and bronze smelters as well as excellent carpenters. From the great forests of Lebanon they took cypress, oak and large sweet-smelling cedar trunks. When king Solomon (10th century B.C.) decided to build the great temple of Jerusalem, he turned to Hiram from Tyros who offered his best carpenters together with gold, silver and precious woods, receiving in trade wheat, oil and wine.

Phoenician ships have been depicted in their entire splendor in historical art. They were traditionally twenty-five meters long; a sail was drawn between two yards and a cable along the axis from stem to stern, to strengthen the cohesion of the planking. There were fifty men crews working the oars, twenty-five men on each side. There were captains, second in commands, a dozen men per ship to make maneuvers and flutists, who set the rhythm for rowing.

The honorary ships were larger than deport ships or military vessels. Heavy and squat, they were called *gauloi* – a Phoenician word meaning round – by ancient writers. They sailed one hundred kilometers per day, relying on the aft wind, but above all, on the energy supplied by the rowers when capricious winds of the Mediterranean were unfavorable. To defend the growing trade routes, the quick witted Phoenician sailors built sleek, fast warships and equipped them with a terrible offensive weapon, the *rostrum* – a bronze harpoon point. The two enormous eyes painted on the bow struck terror in the hearts of their adversaries, but served to show the ship's route. The "trireme" was their most formidable invention. It was 36 meters long, moved by 75 rowers on each side sitting alternatively in file at three overlapping heights. A true queen of the sea, the "trireme" became the symbol of the mortal and terrifying battles that took place at that time on the Mediterranean Sea.

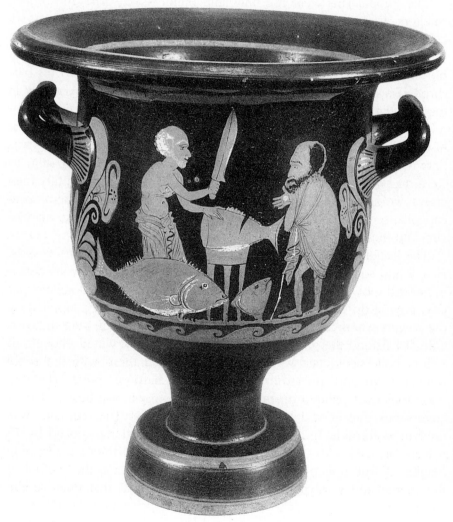

Bell-shaped crater depicting men cutting tuna. 4th century B.C. In the Mandralisca Museum, Cefalù, Sicily.

4 The Greek World

Dining with the gods

Beginning with Homer's description of warrior meals based on bread, grilled meat and wine, all Greek writers concerned themselves with cuisine. Even high on Mt. Olympus among the gods, the favorite pastime was feasting. According to Homer:

> *For the entire day until sunset, they are at the small feast and their hearts have not to complain about a meal in which everyone has taken part. They eat and drink immortal foods, ambrosia and nectar. They listen to music, converse among themselves, they are safe away from the anxieties that men bear upon them.*

Greek cooking brought together the rich culinary delights of severals peoples. There was the well-laid table of the Tarantins, the humble Athenian cuisine, the gluttonous ways of the Boeotians, and the modest cuisine of the Spartans.

Despite the remarkable differences in eating habits between the rich and poor, ancient Greek lifestyle was built on respect for family values and austerity. Although aristocrats had an unpretentious diet, their pantries were full of wine, flour, legumes, dried fruit and oil. They usually ate charcoal-grilled meat on holidays. Meat was expensive and a rare commodity for the underprivileged.

The average Athenian was mostly a vegetarian and ate broad beans, lentils, peas, onions, cabbage, garlic, sea urchins, fried, boiled or roasted fish. The broad beans and lentils were mostly eaten mashed (*etnos*). Athnaios called the Greeks *leaf eaters*; Pláto devoured the sacred olives and was fond of onions; Aristotle was mad about pears and figs.

They also ate poultry, pork, roast beef, mixed stew meats and many eggs. Fowl was in great demand, and always available thanks to the geographical location of the many islands and shaded plains. In the words of Teleclides:

Roasted thrushes with honeyed canapé enter your mouth in a single gulp.

Fish was a very sought after food. Several varieties were used, depending on the economic standing of the consumer. Every solid food accompanied by bread was called *opson*. This included vegetables, onions, olives, meat, fish, fruit and cakes. As time passed, this term came to be used specifically for fish; in modern Greek, the word fish comes directly from *opson*. They ate both fresh and salt-water fish, such as tuna, crab and lobster, clams and mussels, cuttlefish and squid.

Together with bread, fish was everyone's main food. They prepared it in various ways. One recipe that has survived the ages provides instructions on how to cook it in a paper bag. It details cooking slices of "boulter" wrapped in fig leaves. Fish, just as meat, was sold salted or smoked by merchants trading in pickled foods (*tarichos*).

Fishing was a noble trade. Plato wrote the following:

Friends, would that you never lose your taste and pleasure for salt water fishing or for the hook or for any technique used to capture aquatic animals, not even for the lazy fishing using traps which do everything for you, while you are sleeping or vigil.

A splendid artistic drawing found on a 5th century cup shows a boy kneeling on a rock overlooking the sea, holding a fishing rod in one hand and a basketful of fish in the other. Fish are painted in the water with a giant squid and braided wicker basket fish trap; perfect to catch unsuspecting fish that are unfortunate enough to enter.

Wheat was a very precious cereal that the Greeks loved to chew whole and toasted; thus Homer's reference to human "flour eaters." Cereals were the food staple for Athens. From Plato's Republic:

For nourishment men will prepare flour to be toasted or kneaded from barley or wheat, they will make it into beautiful biscuits and breads to serve on strew or well cleaned leaves.

Barley flour kneaded into hardtack (*maza*) cost less than whole wheat bread made into round loaves (*aros*) and was eaten every day. Barley flour was cooked on hot stones or beneath charcoal ashes to make *focaccia* bread that was soft when warm and hard when cool. Whole wheat bread was only eaten on holidays. Hardtack made from barley or wheat could be used as plates, although the Greeks did use plates and bowls made of wood, terracotta or metal to eat puree or boiled dishes. The Greeks spiced their buns and loaves with cumin seeds, sesame seeds and linseed. There were an infinity of breads, from saffron, fennel, rosemary, olive, lard, anise, raisin, capper, sage, garlic, onion, honey, egg, and sweet marjoram. Athenaeum mentioned seventy-two names of bread.

The farmers got most of their energy from a handful of olives with barley or whole wheat bread dipped in wine. The best olives were from Sicione, near Corinth. Already in the 5th century B.C. the Greeks cooked olives in a pan or stored them in brine, in oil and salt, or in seawater called swimming olives (*kolymbades*). Besides *focaccia* bread, made with crushed olives or onions, also stewed and mashed legumes seasoned with olive oil abounded on the table of the general populace. Still today, one of the typical dishes of Puglia, Italy, is puree of dried broad beans seasoned with olive oil.

The day was organized around mealtimes. Breakfast (*acrastima*) was barley or wheat bread soaked in pure wine. It was a light meal that was sometimes enriched with olives or figs. At lunchtime (*arista*), which took place around midday or early afternoon, they prepared legume soup and ate vegetables. The Greeks ate many vegetables. Their principal beverage was wine. Some people ate a very quick snack in the evening (*esperisma*). Supper (*deipna*) was a big hot meal of shellfish or fish, vegetables and barley porridge.

After dinner, at least in homes of the upper-bracket, they washed their hands in bowls of scented water placed on the table (*chernips*) and lost themselves in the pleasures of good wine, salty foods, cheese, black olives and fruit.

The Greeks were always ready for a good meal, but diets were also very successful. Remedies suggested by Galen, a doctor who lived in the 2nd century A.D., were in fact famous. He prescribed a diet rich in vegetables and fish, with olive oil as a seasoning.

Hippocrates, the greatest physician of his time and father of current dieting, considered every food a factor of health or a cause of disease. Heavy foods, in Hyppocrates' opinion, produced black bile that accumulated in the spleen. Foods such as aged cheese, lentils, some thick wines and oversalted meats were to be avoided. Better to eat nutritious foods of wheat, fresh cheese, milk, young meat and broad beans. Besides its intrinsic nutritional value, food had particular virtues. Most vegetables created a refreshing and relaxing effect, carrots and celery were diuretics, red wine was an astringent, apple juice was good for

A person seated before a table of food. Terracotta from the 6th century B.C. In the Louvre, Paris.

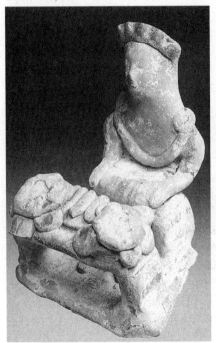

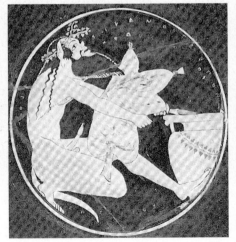

Cup by the Epeleios Painter: the satyr Terpon proclaims that the wine is sweet (hedus hoinos). *Wine for immediate use was placed in skins. End of the 6th century B.C. In the Antikensammlungen, Munich.*

the throat. Fasting was a cure-all for fever, according to the following aphorism:

The more you feed impure bodies, the more damage you cause.

Among the Greeks, *garum* (fish sauce) did not have the fame bestowed upon it by other peoples (Romans and Carthaginians). Ancient processing plants were reported in Corinth and Delos. It is likely that dishes were seasoned only with olive oil, as they still are in this Mediterranean region.

A frequently eaten food by Greek farmers was *kykeon*, something between a solid food and a drink. This ritual drink of the Eleusinian Mysteries was a mixture of barley flour and water, spiced with mint or thyme; it was considered a food with medical properties, as indicated in Aristophanes' Peace, where Trigeus, fearing indigestion from fruit, is given advice to drink kykeon, by Hermes. However, because it was looked upon as peasant food, it was disdained by high society.

Meals often ended with dessert (*tragèma*), consisting of fresh or dried fruit; mostly figs, nuts and grapes or sweets, above all honey. For the Athenians, honey was ambrosia of the gods. Zeus was fed on honey from birth, because no other food could be compared to it. Bees placed honey on Plato's lips and the words leaving his mouth were marvelously sweet, enlightening and, like a thin penetrating perfume emanating from genius, they enchanted the ear and spirit of men.

The Greeks ate many sweets, far more so than the Romans. There were cakes (*placentae*) and different kinds of pastry. There were the ancient *encythus* that had a spiral shape. These were fried in lard. One kind of sweet (*enkrides*) was the precursor of Italian *struffoli*. They even enjoyed apple fritters. Sweet dough was generally made with barley, wheat, rice and sesame seed flours, sweet wine and cheese. Honey was always a main ingredient.

Water was the favored drink of the Greeks, though they also drank milk and a kind of apple juice – a mixture of water and apples. Beer was also known. Xenophon speaks of it in the 4th book of Hellenics:

> *There was also wheat, barley, legumes and barley beer saved in jars containing floating barley grains. Various sized cane straws without knots were also immersed in them. Whenever someone got thirsty he had to take a straw and suck. The drink was too strong when not cut with water, but once tasted it was very good.*

Wine was the more sought after drink. To guarantee the preservation they added salted water or other ingredients, often spices such as thyme, mint or cinnamon, sometimes honey. Wine preservation changed according to where it was produced. In order to be drunk immediately, wine was poured into goat or pigskins, while that for exportation was stored in large terracotta jars (*pithoi*), later to be transferred to clay amphoras lined with resin. Wine was marked by indicating the merchant's name and the names of local magistrates to indicate its origin. The wines from Taso and Chios were famous. Wine exportation was regulated by law, and protected by strict sanctions.

Wine was not drunk straight (*acratos*). They watered it down to create a more or less alcoholic mixture in large clay or wood containers called craters, or smaller easily carried vessels (*oinochoai*).

Greeks served wine above all at banquets. The word symposium literally means a reunion of drinkers. The reunion always began with a meal, and ended with drinking, mostly wine. Many games, dancing and music brightened the atmosphere. At such events wine often went with sweets (*tragemata*), dried or fresh fruit, or broad beans to increase one's thirst. Thus, most feasts ended in general drunkenness.

While feasting, the Greeks loved to eat while lying down with their legs up on the bed with their bodies slightly inclined and held up by pillows. The tables were small and movable. Such information can be gathered from depictions on bas-reliefs or paintings regarding scenes of symposiums. At feasts, both men and women became skilled at *kottabos*. Drinkers enjoyed hitting a target with the dregs of wine remaining at the bottom of the cup while pronouncing the name of the person they desired. Hitting a certain plate or wine vase was a sign that the love story would come true.

Crete, the happy island

"Broad Crete," is how Homer described it, together with the following words:

> *Far away, on the blue sea, lies a land called Crete, a rich and beautiful land, bathed all around by waves, heavily populated, boasting of ninety cities. Each of its many races has its own language... One of the ninety cities is a large metropolis called Cnossus and there, for nine years king Minos reigned over Crete, the happy island, enjoying the friendship with the omnipotent Zeus.*

Crete, so noble among the Mediterranean islands, cradle of Western Civilization, was the site upon which a people between 3400 and 1200 B.C. dominated the seas and ocean commerce. As Aristotle observed:

> *The position of Crete is remarkably beautiful. It dominates the sea around which all the Greeks live... This is why Minos has the thalassocracy and conquered and colonized the island.*

Crete was the first true thalassocracy of the Mediterranean.

Kings and their families lived in palaces with large airy rooms on several floors, situated around a central courtyard. Just as today in that part of the world, the roofs were flat. They used plumbing, drains emptied through the walls. There were toilets and running water and fixed bathtubs made out of baked clay. Little is known about the poor because their houses were generally meager and did not last long.

The Minoan diet was very similar to the current diet on Crete. This is an excellent example of continuous culinary unity for millennia. Most of their meat consisted of pork, mutton and goat. Like today, beef was rare, given the unsuitable Cretian countryside. The land was instead rich in wild game such as deer, boar, hare, duck, goose, and partridge.

Fish was widely eaten and plentiful, as today. They also ate shellfish, clams and octopus. These are still today considered delicious foods.

Bread was made from barley or wheat and probably, like Arab bread today, unrisen. There was also milk from sheep or goats and cheese; butter was unknown.

Fruit was plentiful. They had apples, pears, grapes, pomegranates, figs and dates, and different kinds of nuts. Among the legumes, peas and lentils came first. Olives were the foundation upon which Crete was built. Olive oil was, and still is today a vital part of the diet in these regions. For sweetening they used honey, as there was no sugar.

The leading beverage was wine, but it is likely that the inhabitants also drank tea with the variety of herbs that bloom on Crete.

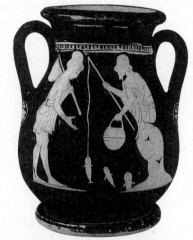

Fixed stoves were a rarity. Cooking was usually done on portable charcoal grills. A remarkable number of copper pots have been found in the palaces and large estates, while the general populace used terracotta tableware, drinking glasses – like our tea cups or our wine glasses – bowls, wine pitchers and jugs. They preferred to store liquids in stirrup jars, with a false spout on top, strap handles on the sides and the working spout. These came in different sizes, starting at just a few centimeters tall and reaching half a meter and more.

Top. Red-figured pelike by the Pan Painter with fishing scenes. Last quarter of the 5th century B.C. In the Kunsthistorisches Museum, Vienna.

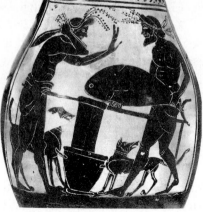

Olpe by the Leagros Group: fish sacrifice. 520 B.C. In the Staatliche Museen, Berlin.

Production goods were deposited in storage rooms within the buildings, and the buildings themselves were art boutiques and even trading centers. The range of trade gives witness to the Minoan works of art found in Egypt, Syria and Cyprus as much as Egyptian, Babylonian art works found in Cretian palaces. One hundred and fifty man-sized *pitoi*, have been found in the Cnossus palace: they contained oil, perhaps even wine and had a capacity of around 78,000 liters. Lead-lined crypts to hold liquids have been brought to light.

The community meal (*andreion*) had an almost institutional importance in ancient Crete. The daily presence at the community table was part of the obligations required to become a citizen and to maintain citizenship. There was also a contribution of raw materials. This was a privilege granted to a limited number of adult men. The community meal was also where young Cretians were educated by listening to the feats of their ancestors, by being reminded of the inferiority of all those unlike themselves. Plutarch reminds us that the community meal as a school persisted in Sparta:

> *The children often came to observe these meals; they were conducted like a school of self-control; there they heard politics discussed, and observed enjoyment fit for free men.*

The mythical Crete of Minotaur, Theseus and Daedalus continues to produce discrete amounts of oil, grapes, cereals, fruit and modern vegetables; gifts of a land facing the wine dark sea.

Sparta, the austere cuisine

The egalitarian idea of the reformer Lycurgus even upset the community table of the Spartans. It was not enough that the society had culturally reached a plateau, and evidence that a better society had not been obtained was worthless. It was taken into little consideration that the wealth had slipped out of the city that had become a sanctuary for impoverished citizens. The Spartans had to eat at the same community table, partake of the same food, be perhaps obliged to demonstrate the mouthfuls taken to avoid the punishment of those who would dare to break the culinary rules.

Exasperated egalitarianism, it is known, does not benefit the cuisine. And so the poor Spartan resigned to look at the famous or ill-famed black soup, the recipe we choose to ignore. It was perhaps a sort of dense stew with ingredients such as pork, blood, vinegar and salt.

Fortunately, cheese, together with barley and figs, were there to give some variety to Spartan communal meals. Cheese was always eaten in its natural state, so they must have envied cheeses blended with a large number of ingredients, among which honey. These were true delicacies for those lucky enough to have enjoyed them.

Plutarch tells us that the king of Pontus was curious to taste the famous black soup and so hired a Spartan cook to prepare it for him. The king, however, found it horrid. The cook gave the following comment:

> *Your Majesty, this food should be eaten after bathing in the Eurota river.*

It is likely that the Spartans bathed before eating, not only to compensate for their scarce contact with water or for reasons of hygiene, but perhaps to better appreciate the hot soup.

The Spartan wooden or metal drinking cups (*cothon*) were not well finished. Plutarch pointed out:

> *The lacquer covering blocked the distinction of dirty water that the soldiers were forced to drink and would have disgusted them. Moreover, the mud that dirtied the water was held back at the inside rim of the cup and the water thus arrived at the mouth cleaner.*

In a society nourished on black soup and thirst quenched with impure water, it was no wonder that the hard natural selection allowed only the strongest, perhaps also the most stupid, to literally stay alive. The myth of the tough Spartan, tempered to serve his country, was fed by anecdotes of ignorant soldiers. During one banquet, for example, a Spartan guest was given a sea urchin to eat. He had never before heard of such a thing. "What am I to do with that black pointy thing?" he asked. He remained clueless, but undaunted. A lot of chewing seemed to be the solution. Unfortunately, the job turned out to be harder than he had figured. At the height of his desperation for the insult he had received at a foreigner's table, the distressed Spartan exclaimed:

Foul mouthful! Do not think that I would be cowardly enough to spit it out. Rest assured that you will not trick me again.

This is a typically tough attitude.

Feasts, symposiums and guests

Family get-togethers, community holidays and all the events considered worthy of celebration – the coming or going of family and friends, winning sports events or poem contests – ended in a feast.

The terms banquet, symposium, or feast were generally used as synonyms, although there are differences, perhaps slight but symbolic for a Greek way of thinking. Every banquet for a festivity, religious brotherhood, social or sports event, was broken up into two parts: the first filled the stomach and alleviated hunger; the second involved drinking wine and playing a variety of games that warmed the atmosphere and made the hosts and guests merry. These were literally drinking parties, where each person was called upon to speak on a given topic.

Those who organized the banquet in their own homes invited those they met in the Agora or on the street, and never denied attendance to a friend of a friend. At the same time they tried to identify the usual parasite attempting to only scrounge a meal. The host waited for his guests in the *andron*, a room reserved for men and feasts. Once their shoes were removed, and their feet washed, the invited guests reclined on *klinai*, rectangular beds where they rested with their bodies slightly inclined and held up by rich pillows designed with geometric patterns. Below the bed a hanger held footwear. Two or three guests shared each bed, and every bed supported a small rectangular table upon which previously prepared portions of food were served in vessels and plates. The guests often wore leaf and flower crowns.

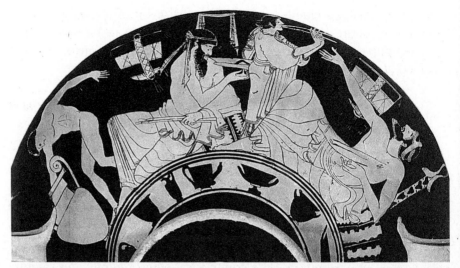

Red-figured cup attributed to Douris, depicting the pleasures of the feast: music, games and drinking. Beginning of the 5th century B.C. In the Vatican Museums, Vatican City.

The habit of washing their hands in a basin brought around by slaves was necessary in absence of forks. Finally, they passed around the cup filled with *pronoma*, a spiced wine that warmed the heart and wet the appetite. On the table, trays held neatly arranged terracotta plates containing appetizers such as garlic, sea urchins, hot *focaccia* bread, shellfish, pieces of sturgeon, and a heaping of vegetables. All these delicacies were necessary to moderately enhance taste, while waiting for Chios wine that the owner carefully decanted and that a slave mixed with water in large craters. The cups of those attending the feast were filled from small vessels (*oinochoai*). The hard-working slaves poured the wine. The household dogs, used to such customs, already began to move about under the beds in search of breadcrumbs used to clean hands and thrown onto the floor.

The chef had received instructions from the patron to restrict the menu to just fish, because that evening some learned men would be attending the symposium and the guests had to remain rather sober to discuss the topics to be chosen. Visiting the fish market, the chef had purchased a beautiful, still throbbing boulter.

Once the boulter was cut into slices and wrapped in fig leaves, it was baked to perfection and now was a sight to behold dressed with green and black olives, vegetables, onions and various legumes. There was little supper for the whining dogs.

For dessert, out came fresh fruits and savory sweets. That evening nothing less than the famous *amphiphos* cake dedicated to Artemides was made. When ringed with crepes and dipped in honey it was a real delicacy. Some guests may have contemplated the poor state of dessert when it consisted only of bay leaves, to be chewed after dinner. But that was only a memory, and it was already fading.

After dessert, came the symposium. Some invited guests took their leave guided by a female flautist cloaked in a vale that left little room for imagination; perhaps she would otherwise have gone to the *gynae-ceum* to perform for the women of the house. All the wives and mothers were banned from the festivities. The flautist would sometimes return to the symposium to accompany other guests that had in the meantime arrived. The musicians, dancers or prostitutes admitted to feasts for their decorative roles had sad destinies. They were considered subhuman. Wanting to or not, they livened up the party, even though, for them, it was merely a way to escape hunger. Menander described it in the following way:

> To earn ten wretched drachmas, certain prostitutes regularly attend the feasts and drink straight wine until they burst or if they do not do so quickly and without turning up their noses, they end up dying of hunger.

Feasts began with libations to Dionysus, the decent god that had donated wine to humanity. Small sips were taken of uncut wine, and a few drops were spilled purposely on the floor, invoking the god. They designated the king of the feast (*symposiarch*) who established the proportion of wine and water to be mixed together and the amount of wine to be drunk.

Some drinkers took delight in hitting a target with the dregs remaining at the bottom of their cups, thus beginning the game of *kottabos*. The game had many variations, but was in principle one of seduction.

Whenever a drop fell on a predetermined object, it was interpreted as a favorable sign regarding a loved one, even fleeting loves whose name was pronounced as the throw was made. To this standard version others soon followed, always with the enthusiasm of a prize.

What prizes could they hope to receive? Eggs, apples, sweets, or sandals, necklaces, ribbons, cups, balls, or more simply, a kiss. To be proclaimed a winner, one had to sink the most terracotta cups floating in a tub of water by hitting them with wine, or cause a plate balanced on a vertical pole to fall and strike an inverted cup attached to the pole two thirds of the way up.

After the 3rd century B.C., *kottabos* fell into disuse. Banquet participants then adopted other games to express their desires. They threw quince apples, that consecrated fruit to Aphrodite, to celebrate the legendary gesture of the shepherd Paris, when he was asked on Mt. Ida to choose the most beautiful of the three gods. The name of the elected was carved on the fruit.

> *I am an apple thrown by the man who loves you. Accept it, Xanthippe.*
> *One day we will both be past our prime.*

No cost was too high for the host to spend on his guests. Four *congi* of pure wine – about thirteen liters – was usual. The Greeks were avid drinkers. All of them, with no exceptions, had to drink until reaching the same degree of inebriation at the symposium. Such

Red-figured cup showing a young man as he vomits into a basin. Late 5th century B.C. In the Vatican Museums, Vatican City.

was the requirement to conduct an intelligent discussion. That was a true democracy.

Symposiums often ended in general drunken abandonment. The dancers who were sometimes a little more sober than the guests held up the men so unrestrained in drinking. The return home must have been a piteous sight.

The cuisine in literature

Gastronomic literature was always considered a humble activity compared to those of more important themes – epics, tragedies, histories – but was nonetheless developed, often with parodistic tones. The referral to hunger, cooking and to red wine were used to their maximum for humor in ancient plays.

The first known cooking school was founded in the 3rd century B.C. by Labdacus in Syracuse – birthplace of Terpsione, founder of the academy which taught the art of serving guests, setting tables and finding just the right match between food and wine. Through written histories we know that Mithecus, another resident of Syracuse and great inventor of dishes and very refined recipes, was to culinary arts what Phidias was in sculpture. Ultimately, Mithecus worked his art in Greece after the fiasco brought upon him by Sparta.

The best known from Syracuse was Archestratus of Gela who in 330 B.C. published *Hedypatheia* (i.e., the pleasure of taste), codifying the principles that are today the very foundation of modern cooking.

Archestratus is reasonably well known because a good part of his writing has come down to us. His philosophy was based on a cardinal idea to save the natural taste of the food and bring out its freshness, without ruining it with sauces, gravies, or overcooking. A very singular passage describes the choice of a marine locality where good fish were found:

> *Everyone raves about the eels, but the best without question is taken in the sea at the straits facing Reggio. There you, Messenio, rise above all other mortal men, placing in your mouth such a food.*

And again:

Eat the best elope preferably in noble Syracuse. Indeed this fish in principle was born there. When fished near the islands or the coast of Asia or Crete it is small, tough, and exhausted by the waves.

The details where various animal or vegetable products come from were also described by Archestratus. Regarding tuna, for example, we have the following:

Very good examples are found even in Bysantium and in Charistus; but on the glorious island of Sicily you find better tuna than these. In fact the tuna that feed along the coast of Cefalù and Tindari are among the best. If however, you find yourself one day in Ippona, illustrious city of the Bruzzi, in Italy, surrounded by water, you will find the best, nor are there others that can compete with them for the record.

Red-figured cup by Makron with a scene of meat being boiled in a cauldron. 490 B.C. In the Louvre, Paris.

Cup from the workshop of the Nikosthenes Painter with a satyr diving into a container of wine. 500 B.C. In the Musée d'Art et d'Histoire, Geneva.

There is also a recipe for hare among this work:

As for the hare, there are many ways and many rules to prepare it; but the best way is to serve it hot to table companions; some roasted meat for everyone to rip from the skewer a little rare with only salt sprinkled on it. It does not disturb you to see the red dripping from the pieces, on the contrary, voraciously eat. For me the other recipes are absolutely excessive, mixing grease with cheese and oil, unrestrained, like one preparing to eat cat.

Archestratus' poem, permeated as it was with affability and humor, was famous in his day. It crossed the boarders of Greece and reached those from other lands.

Ennius, the father of the Latin epic poetry, wrote a cookbook that celebrated refined eating with a title and content in parallel with the one written by Archestratus.

> *Always during the meal encircle your head with different laurels provided by the rich soil of the earth, and fix your hair with pleasant distilled oils, and on live coals sprinkle mirth and incense all day, perfumed product of Syria. When you drink be served a final dish like this: tripe and boiled sow vulva, immersed in cumin and strong vinegar and sylph and tender species of roasted birds in season; do not bother that those from Syracuse only drink like frogs, without eating anything.*

Other masters of gastronomy were Aegis from Rodes, Nereus from Chios, a fish expert, Carydes from Athens, famous for his Tyron pudding. This is how the comic poet Antiphanes makes a the distinction between ancient cooking and that in vogue (4th century B.C.):

> *Here is where we have arrived! Bread, garlic, cheese, maza, these yes are healthy foods, instead of the salting of fish, the lamb chops dusted with spices, the sweet mixtures, and the corrupting prostitute stews. And what shall we say of the cabbages cooked over a slow fire in oil, for Zeus, and eaten with pea puree.*

Perhaps Teleclides, a comic author from the 5th century B.C., said it best when he gave a voice to Crhonos, father of Jove, of the good times passed and gone, of the mythical age of gold, where abundance reigned, denied to men after the Prometheus outrage:

> *The first thing was peace for all as there is water for the hands. The earth produced neither terror nor disease and foods appeared spontaneously. The streams flowed with wine. Barley and wheat bread competed in front of the mouths of men begging to be swallowed if they loved white*

bread. Fish came into houses, fried and served themselves at the table. A river of soup ran beside the beds, carrying pieces of hot meat. Canals full of spicy gravy were there for those who wanted it, without the bother of dipping a morsel and swallowing a tender mouthful. In bowls sweets dusted with spices appeared. Roasted larks accompanied with milk biscuits flew down your throat and the focaccia *breads moved in a warrior's tumult around the jaws. The children played knucklebones with delicate pieces of sow vulva and delicacies. In those times men were large, enormous giants.*

5 The misteriuos Etruscans

Dining with the Lucumons

A very ancient people, like no others in language or customs.

That is how Dionysius of Halicarnassus defined the Etruscans, a people with the gift of popular wisdom and good taste in observation and expression.

The Etruscans have always inspired the creators of myth, in which truth became mixed with fantasy. Herodotus tells us the following:

During the reign of Atys, son of Manes (13th century B.C.), a strong famine struck all of Lydia. For a certain period of time the Lydians continued their lifestyle, then attempting to find a remedy to the persistent famine, one after another contemplated. It was then that the game of dice was supposedly invented... Every other day, they played all day long, to ward of the temptation to eat; the day after they left the game and ate. They went on like this for eighteen years. But since the scourge, instead of waning, became ever more violent, the king, after dividing his subjects into two groups, left it to fate which would remain and which would emigrate. He decided not to abandon the group that was destined to stay and put his son Tyrrhenus at the head of the group that had to leave. Those that fate would have it left the country, ... they arrived in Umbria, where they built the city where they still live now. With the desire to change their name with another, derived from the King's son that guided them in their adventure, they adopted Tyrrheni.

The Romans called them *Tusci* (from which we now have the word Tuscany) and *Etrusci* (from which we get the word Etruscans). The tale told by Herodotus, with exception made for legend, found supporters for the hypothesis suggesting the origin of the Etruscans was Asia Minor. This allowed for a better understanding of the oriental features of their civilization and attachment to their fertile land.

The fertility of Etruscan soil was, in fact, highly celebrated by the ancients. Nature offered all its gifts, all the fruit of the land generously repaid the efforts of the farmers. There were abundant crops and grape harvests, strong plants, a fertile country that was well farmed, with plenty of resources and every kind of cultivation. It was an ideal landscape where the grapevine married the olive tree. In this land, corresponding to Tuscany and above all to a vast zone designated by the name of the Etruscan fields, which extended from Fiesole to Arezzo, grew grain, livestock and an array of other foods.

Pliny the Younger wrote the following description to a friend towards the end of the 1st century A.D.:

The landscape is very beautiful. Imagine an immense amphitheater, which only nature can make. A vast and spacious plain with a belt of mountains that have at their tops ancient high trunk woods. The wild game is plentiful and varied, from high up the stands of timber descend in a slope. In the middle, fertile hills covered with good land (since nowhere is it easy to find rock, even if you search for it) no less fertile than the fields situated on the true plains: rich crops that ripen later, it is true, but not less well. At their feet, on every side, vineyards spread out, linked to one another to uniformly cover a far and wide space. At the bottom, almost setting up a boarder, grow woods then grassland and wheat fields, that cannot be ploughed without the help of stout oxen and heavy-duty ploughs... This variety, this happy disposition, wherever you lie your eyes, is heartening.

Some years earlier, Titus Livius described much more fertile and broad Etruscan countryside than the Roman heartland with the following words:

The fields, on the plains and hills, are favored by the healthy climate, there are no swamps nearby, nor are there rivers that can make the air cold in the morning, only pure and plentiful springs.

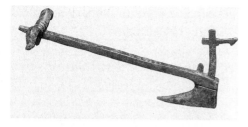

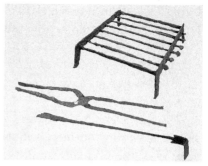

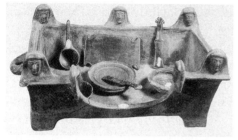

Top left. *Bronze plow, from Talamone. In the Archeology Museum, Florence.*

Top right. *Etruscan cooking utensils, a metal rack and thongs. In the Villa Giulia Museum, Rome.*

Middle left. *Small hearth in bucchero. Second half of the 6th century B.C. In the Archeology Museum, Chiusi.*

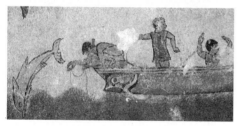

Bottom left. *Hunting and Fishing tomb: fishing with drop-lines, harpoons and nets. Early 6th century B.C. Tarquinia.*

It was this fertile land that grew products eaten on ancient Etruscan tables.

The Etruscan day unfortunately is unknown in all of its details. The only certain thing that has reached us regards the time available to eat two meals a day. Poseidonius of Apamea said:

> *The Etruscans set a sumptuous table twice a day with everything that contributes to a delicate life, they prepare the tablecloth with flower needlepoint, lie out a quantity of silver tableware and are waited on by a considerable number of servants.*

The great organization of the Etruscan kitchen deserves a remark. This has come down to us from scenes depicted above all in room tombs. These are messages of perfect organization in culinary activities, and reflect the gracious government of the Etruscans.

With them it is not only free men, but also most the servants who have every type of single home.

The Etruscans used ovens to cook bread and meat, or portable clay stoves to set in the hearth. Sometimes the hearth took on the appearance of a true fireplace equipped with a hood.

In Golini's tomb at Orvieto, built towards the first half of the 4th century B.C. for the Leinie (Laenii) family, there is a painting of a funeral banquet for two brothers in the presence of Ade and Proserpina. It describes the activity of eleven servants preparing the meal in the kitchen.

The Golini tomb painting shows a *carnarium* with butchered meat and wild game, an entire beef with its head cut off, large eyes worthy of Juno, a hare and a deer hanging between two pairs of fowl, farm animals and wild game together. Bacon – *venter faliscus* as defined by Varro in *De Re Rustica* – was very well liked, as was the famous *lucana* sausage. Even Cecil Statius cites small lard, *lucanica* (sausage) and Etruscan ponderous *ventresche* (heavy Etruscan bacon). As for the processing and cooking, small, cut pieces of meat could be boiled in large bronze caldrons, probably together with legumes and cereals, or roasted on grills or skewered.

Well known, but rarely used, were two sides of beef (*mezzema*) with each half stuffed with herbs, pepper corns, garlic and onions, all basted with wine must or vinegar. Bronze caldrons, grills, skewers and clay stoves have been found deposited in tombs and confirm this way of cooking meat. Eating meat was reserved for sacrificial ceremonies and festivities, at least for the population at large. At a wedding ceremony, for example, Titus Livius refers to the sacrificing of the first born from a herd of pigs.

Just as well known to the Romans was the reputation of *pecorino* cheese, made from the milk of *Luni* sheep on the boarder of Liguria. These were made into gigantic forms of cheese that weighed sometimes as much as a thousand pounds, nearly 327 kilograms of very good *caseus lunensis*, enough for a thousand lunches.

In another tomb scene there is a domestic, perhaps a baker, knead-ing flour. The tools in his hands make you think more of cutting than kneading dough for the preparation of one of those elaborate dishes that made the ancients gluttonous. Every kind of ingredient was includ-ed, carefully chopped, and heavily spiced. Chopped cereals or legumes, but also seeds, herbs and essences, were required to prepare the meat seasonings. As a matter of fact, in the Moretum, attributed to Virgil, a farmer prepares a shepherd's pie made of herbs, garlic, cheese and wine in a mortar with a small pestle. Apicius, the Brillat Savarin of Rome during the reign of Tiberius, whose name was found even in a Cere tomb, passed down a recipe with the secret of knowing how to finely chop (*terere*). This was so important in preparing hare gravy with peppercorns, privet (*levisticum* or *ligustrum*), celery seeds, garum, silphium, and a touch of wine and oil.

The Etruscans loved to cook to the sound of music. To set the rhythm for the grinder, a *tibicen* called Tr. Thun Suplu played for him. Tr. is likely an abbreviation for Trepu or Trebius. Thun is the relation-ship of the name with the ordinal number 1 and perhaps means *primus*. Suplu is certainly the same word as *subulo*, which Varro tells us was the Etruscan name of the flute player.

The enormous importance attributed to music in the life of the Etruscans is certainly one of the most extraordinary features of their civilization. With the following words, Aristotle mentioned that he was aware of how the Etruscans lived:

> *The Etruscans boxed, whipped servants and cooked to the sound of flute, which leads one to surmise that all daytime jobs, even the most banal, were carried out to the beat of music.*

And he believed it to be a sign of laziness. Silence must have been difficult to find in an Etruscan city.

Continuing our detailed examination of the wall in Golini's tomb, we recognize a miniature stove with two half-naked servants. A servant girl, Thrama Mlithuns, is there and, with a gesture, invites Thresu F. Sithrals, who brings a table to the guests' bed. Piles of *focaccia* breads, probably round, other foodstuffs, eggs, clusters of dark grapes are depicted on the rectangular three-legged table, in the Greek manner that has spread throughout Etruria. However, sitting in a pile of grapes one can also see a pomegranate flanked by two small pyramids, or so it seems, of sweets. The tomb also contains a painting of another aspect of servitude. On a wooden table there are all types of trays, every kind of small dark purple container, long stemmed cups, glasses, large bowls that seem to be filled with a yellow or reddish substance. You can also see bronze carafes, perhaps a *kylix* with large handles capped by a cover with a spout. It reminds one of certain vases in the Apulian style of southeastern Italy.

In an inscription from Falerii, using an archaic and dialect Latin, he jokingly boasts of the culinary value of their trade:

> *Quei soueis argutiais opidque Volcani condecorant saipisume comvivia loidosque (With their wit and help from Vulcan, they confer all of their splendor to banquets and the games).*

If the Sybarites braided crowns for their cooks, the Etruscans must not have held them in any less regard.

An important place at the ancient Etruscan table was taken by wine. Etruscan wines were known in Greece: Dionysius of Halicarnassus considered them generally as equal to Falernum. In cisalpine Gaul they celebrated the wines from Adria, Cesena and a Maecenatianum, produced on the property of Mecenatus. An excellent wine came from the Graviscae vineyards. From the Veio territory came a light rosé and was enjoyed only by the purses of frugal landlords.

The Etruscans preferred muscat, the sweet taste of which, they said, caused the bees (*apes*) to be gluttonous. They thus called them *Apianae* wines, sweet wines that went to one's head. This was the wine drunk by those attending banquets, as captured in paintings. All these varieties denote the long experience of the Etruscan people in wine making.

The drinking of wine is one of the more important scenes in Etruscan depictions, particularly in those found in the tombs. Also found in these burial sites were utensils such as ladles, strainers, and pitchers used mostly for wine. Wine became *keimelion*, that is to say, a

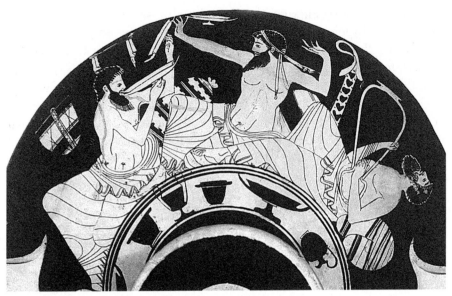

Red-figured cup attributed to Douris, depicting the pleasures of the feast: music, games and drinking. Beginning of the 5th century B.C. In the Vatican Museums, Vatican City.

prestigious commodity, a noble and precious beverage. Such importance of wine can be understood even from its scarce representation at meals. The tomb of the Scudi at Tarquinia (350-325 B.C.) depicts courses of *focaccia* breads and vegetables but no wine.

Etruscan vegetable gardens were known for their legumes. Authors of antiquity boasted of the Ariccia leeks, the turnips from Nursia, the onions from Tuscolo and the asparagus from Ravenna. From floral decorations of funeral paintings and art work not taken from the oriental repertory, one can recognize artichokes, convolvulus, ivy, dwarf palm and the oak as part of the local flora, as well as acanthus, bay leaf, cypress, lily, poppy, and pomegranate. The latter appears at Cere on plaques painted in the 6th century B.C. The Punic apple (*malum punicum*) is supposed to have been discovered by the Carthaginians. According to Pliny the Elder, the turnip held third place among the more remunerative products for commercial trade, right after grapes and wheat. But broad beans also held a high place because without them, Pliny tells us nothing was done in the kitchen.

Etruria produced enough cereals to be able to export them to near-by countries. Spelt came from Chiusi. It is remembered for the white-ness of its flour (*candoris nitidi*), which Ovid recommended to his readers to use as facial powder. It also served to prepare *focaccia* bread (*clusinae pultes*). For the longest time, this was the main nutrient of the Etruscans and Italics. Chiusi and Arezzo were also famous for their common wheat, the "siligo", used to make refined bread. What we call pasta was also very renowned. This was made with a type of wheat durum (*alica*) mixed with wine and honey. Cisalpine Gaul was particularly suitable to grow millet.

The amount of Etruscan food deposits that have come to light, with wheat, cereals and legumes, furnishes direct proof that their diet was based, perhaps as in Rome, on *puls*, a type of mush made with spelt flour kneaded with water. This provided enough calories for survival. Moreover, the consistency of leguminous plants demonstrates how already widespread was the practice of the fallow field, in which legumes rotated with grain to allow a continuous tillage of the earth for future seeding.

Spelt (dressed wheat) was certainly the most important cereal in Etruria. It was more widely used because it was tougher and stood up better to the cold winters. The roasting was an important moment in its treatment because it eliminated glume and water. It was so impor-tant that during Numa Pompilius' time a festival was celebrated in honor of the kiln. The kiln then was elected to be a god, with the hope that it would intercede to end the fires that started by burning spelt directly over the flames. Many authors have reported Rome's reliance on massive grain imports from Etruria. At least three times in the 5th century B.C. large quantities of cereal were imported as quick-ly as possible because of famine. At the end of the 2nd century B.C., according to Titus Livius, the Etruscans furnished Scipio Africanus wheat and supplies destined for the Roman fleet engaged in the second Punic war (205 B.C.):

> Cere gave wheat and every kind of foodstuff... Volterra furnished grain...Arezzo 100 bushels of wheat... Perugia, Chiusi and Roselle a great quantity of wheat.

The feasts

Feasts were important in Etruscan life. Numerous portrayals on sarcophaguses and ash urns, but above all the paintings in the room tombs at Tarquinia, Chiusi and Orvieto, describe scenes of food eaten while reclining on a couch, scenes of dancing and banquets running over with wine, cups of wine and ladles with which to pour it. Such feasts became almost ritual.

The splendid fresco paintings in the Tarquinia tombs are modeled in bas-relief on terracotta from Velletri, and sculptured on urns and memorial stones from Chiusi. There one can see the couch taken up by two guests, the small table before the bed, a rooster or dog beneath the table, musicians playing a double flute and a designated wine servant filling the cups. This was a way to relate daily life, as well as to flaunt status, the social standing of the deceased.

The tableware used by the guests was plentiful and varied. They utilized small buckets, basins, pitchers, bowls, and cups, sometimes decorated with incisions or relief. These objects adorned the princely tombs of the 7th century B.C. at Vetulonia, Cere or Preneste. In one of the frescos in the Tomb of the Painted Vases at Tarquinia (end of the 6th century B.C.), a large white *kylix*, perhaps made of silver, is depicted in the hands of a feast-goer. The vases generally depicted at banquets were made of ceramic or bronze.

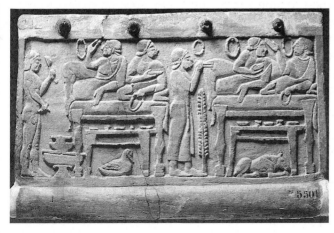

Ionic-Etruscan style relief sculpture from Chiusi. A feast with a flute player, a servant and animals under the tables. Half of the 6th century B.C. In the Archeology Museum, Florence.

Nothing can be said about the place and time of these feasts. They occurred in an imaginative setting. In the Leopards' tomb, the young banqueters crowned with mirth are lost in the careless pleasures of wine and lust for women. The men, with dark hair, while the women with blond hair are all dressed in splendid multicolored capes. The couple in the foreground fix their gaze on a Ganymede passing nude before them with a pitcher. There is tickling, small talk, and waves of desire.

The scenes depicted with so many festivities, painted with such lively colors, show a serene lifestyle that will not survive the coming of the Hellenistic world when feasts will be dedicated to gods beyond the grave, at times repelling, other times attractive, but always bathed in gloom and never merry. The scenes of daily life painted on the walls often seem to take place in the open, among complaisant shrubs and buildings, perhaps the hunt. The household animals are pictured contemplating the leftovers of the feast, while the servants are ready for every beck and call. The atmosphere is enlivened by dancers and jugglers. These are uses and customs of a people sealed on the walls to perpetuate the memory to the living and dead.

Etruscan women were allowed to attend feasts, a liberty not given to Greek women. In Athens only courtesans reclined on couches at the table beside young men. In the tomb of the Scudi at Tarquinia, from the 3rd and maybe 2nd century B.C., Velia Seitithi is seated humbly at the feet of the couch next to the crowned Larth Velcha.

Unlike their Roman counterparts, Etruscan women had a given name and saved the surnames of both parents, thus completing their full name. This rule carried for women of noble standing, such as Tanaquilla, bride of Tarquin Priscus. The Etruscan woman was queen of her home, within a society that was far from being matriarchal, and differed greatly from that of the androcentric Greeks and Romans.

Under the influence of oriental fashion, the lifestyle of the nuclear family was transformed. Women, attended by servants, were assigned the task of setting up the feast. Although they had to continue work at the loom, as documented by archaeological findings, women took part at feasts and spectacles. They also shared decisions with their husbands.

These aspects of the Etruscan society suggested a distorted vision of women to Theopompus, a Greek writer from the 4th century B.C. He saw them as rude careless drinkers who were excessively free. An Etruscan woman who took part in daily events was aware of her role as wife. She worried about her beauty, using waxes, oils and perfumes, mostly imported from the Orient and from the Aegean basin. She would have her hair done with clips, possess a rich collection of toiletries consisting of combs, pins, nail cleaners, and mirrors (starting in the 6th century B.C.). The Etruscan wife would use clay basins for the bath (as those found at Marzabotto), and wear jewelry, among which the never lacking buckle to hold cloths, bracelets, earrings and diadems.

Also, because of their refinement, the fondness of the Etruscans for sweets remained legendary among the Romans, as well as the unavoidable corpulence that followed the feasts of meat after the sacrifices:

> *Etruscan fat* (Virgil), *obese Etruscan* (Catullus), *fatter than the flutist* (Servius), *all mush and fat* (Plautus).

Hunting and fishing

Etruria, so rich in woodland, hills, plains, carpeted with forests and shrubs, was ideal for hunters using bow, spear and snare nets to chase deer, boar and water fowl. Every form of wildlife was represented on monuments together with weapons, pikes, javelins and axes, hounds on the trail of prey, the horn in the deep woods, and the return from the hunt. In the scribbling of the Certosa *situla* and on paintings in the Querciola and Scrofa Nera tombs at Tarquinia, scenes of boar hunts, deer hunting and hare hunts are portrayed as part of the Etruscan lifestyle.

Etruscan art had taste for certain decorative animal figures. Although real wolves roamed the land, the matching panthers on a column, lions leaping on gazelles, sphinxes and griffins were pure illusion. A very well known tomb in Chiusi dating to the first half of the 5th century B.C. shows funeral games with all the attractions of a popular circus, while a monkey chained between a dwarf and tightrope walker of the company looks on.

Birds that the haruspex studied were often present in Etruscan art. Prediction books (*Ostentaria*) were illustrated with species and descriptions that gave meaning to an omen. It is to these texts that we owe our knowledge of the Etruscan names for the eagle (*antar*), the sparrow hawk (*arac*), and the falcon (*capu*).

In Etruscan paintings there are many splendid birds represented in full flight or searching for food among the trees. Triclinio's tomb is a true aviary where, without counting the rooster and the hen threatened by a cat under the feast couch, the dancers zigzag through blackbirds and thrushes perched on branches. Thrushes and pheasants were considered real delicacies of the Etruscan kitchen. Browned thrushes basted with honey, boiled and roasted pheasant, all accompanied by fermented milk and raisin wine made for hearty eating and festivities.

Strabo noted that waterfowl was one of the Etruscan wetland attractions. In the haruspex scene of the François tomb one can recognize a woodpecker ready for flight.

Music played an important role in hunting. In *The History of Animals*, written in the 2nd century A.D. by Elianus, music was used to attract game into nets:

> *A story, often remembered by the Etruscans, pretends that in their land, boar and deer get captured not only with snares and gods, in the usual way, but with the help of music. Here is how – they take their nets and other hunting gear and set their traps for game; but then out jumps a talented flutist, who tries to play the most harmonious melodies or replay all the sweetest flute music. In the general peace and quiet this music reaches the*

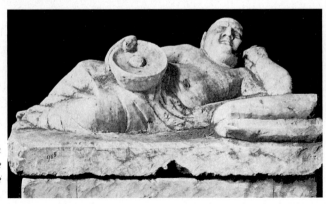

An obese Etruscan: an ash cover in the image of the defunct. In the Etruscan Museum, Chiusi.

shores, the valleys and at the bottom of the forests the sound, to say it in a word, penetrates all the animal hiding places dens. They are first surprised and frightened; then the pure and irresistible pleasure of the music overwhelms them, and when they get curious they forget their young and their dens. Although the animals are not fond of distancing themselves from their lairs, they get drawn along as if a spell is cast over them, under the wonder of the melody, they get close and fall into the snares of the hunters, victims of the music.

The written texts are limited in regards to fishing, telling only of tuna harvests. There are two *thynnoscopes* or observation points on the promontories of Populonia and Mt. Argentario above Orbetello where Etruscans watched for the arrival of schools. We also know that they stocked the lakes of Bracciano, Bolsena and Vico with pike, gilthead and various species of salt water fish that acclimatized to fresh water, and that Pirgi, the port of Cere, was likewise famous for its fishing.

The use of fish in the Etruscan diet has been confirmed by frequent portrayals of typical fish products from the Tyrrheanian Sea, recognizable in fish dishes of the 4th-2nd century B.C., in numerous fishing gear found in tombs, hooks, weights for nets, har-

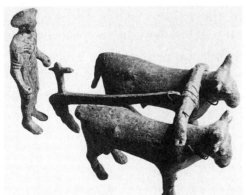

Fish-plate. Second half of the 4th century B.C. In the Archeology Museum, Cerveteri.

Left. *Votive bronze cast of a farmer, from Arezzo. End of the 5th century B.C. In the Villa Giulia Museum, Rome.*

poons, and the remains of seafood. In Verrucchio's tomb, dating to the 7th century B.C., archaeologists have found the remains of a funeral meal consisting of hare bones and a long fish bone in hemispheric terracotta bowls. We can surmise that the meal was accompanied by wine from the presence of a complete set of terracotta bowls, and by grape seeds and hazelnuts.

Of all the tombs discovered in the eighteenth century, one in particular stands out. This tomb has two rooms with splendid paintings of hunting and fishing. In the first room small trees symmetrically outline the space where colored ribbons appear and on the fronton there is a hare hunt. Men on horses advance behind hounds and men beating the ground, while the frightened prey hides behind a bush hoping to escape the destiny that has already befallen the animals carried on the back of servants bringing up the rear.

The second room is frescoed with a scene bathed in particular light. Small boats with fishermen sail on a sea filled with fish, while birds in flight balance above the heads of the busy fishermen. At the center of the adjoining wall a diver jumps from a cliff and dives into the water. A companion is seen climbing the cliff and getting ready to follow him into the wavy sea, rough from the dolphins and waterfowl.

On the fronton of the wall close to the bottom there is a man and woman at a feast, reclining on pillows and seeking each other's eyes while speaking. In the background, a flutist plays and a servant runs to fill cups from large tubs. In the opposite corner two young girls bow on their flower crowns.

This place destined to receive the remains of the deceased was bathed in a serene atmosphere that had to offer a happy picture of the life just left.

6 Rome, caput mundi

Dinner with Lucullus

Two small meals, one very frugal (even only a glass of water) at day-break (*jentaculum*); the second between 11:00 o'clock a.m. and 12:00 noon (*prandium*). Finally, a third more copious meal (*coena*) was eaten at the end of the work day, between 4:00 and 6:00 o'clock p.m.

Pliny the Elder tells us that around 280 B.C. the only important meal was dinner, composed of hot minestrone, the *puls*, a sort of flour polenta cooked in boiling water, followed by cheese, wild game or fish. During the day they ate barley or wheat bread with olives and cheese frugally, on their feet and *sine mensa* (without a table).

Besides what has been written by Latin authors, even figurative art-work competed to mark the boundaries of our knowledge of ancient Roman eating habits. Particularly, some mosaics show the remains of foods that were thrown on the floor during banquets: one of the most famous by Sosus from Pergamum, held the design of chicken bones, fish bones, eggshells, fruit peels, seashells and crab pincers. These table scraps would have been washed away with water. Archeological findings have offered a global view of the kitchen utensils used by the Romans. They were similar to those of modern times: pots, colanders, bread and cake pans, baking pans, frying pans, graters, skewers and many drinking vessels.

Roman eating habits went through several changes over time, thanks above all to contact made with peoples from different cultures. All this brought about different ways to satisfy the pleasures of dining. Horace tells us, with usual irony, that transitory fashions and whims so influenced the golden youth of Rome that it became overwhelmingly disgraceful. The simple cooking of the ancient Romans, rich in flour products and vegetables and with unsophisticated seasonings, such as salt, vinegar, oil and wine, had been transformed by the 1st century A.D. into a refined cuisine, with precious fowl and snails at rich household banquets.

Lucullan feasts, remembered for the choice dishes served during unending dinners, were already a reality in the 1st century B.C. General Lucius Licinius Lucullus who later acquired great wealth, was no slouch: he innovated fisheries, imported cherries to Italy from the Asian city of Cerasonte (hence Cerasum or cherry tree) in 73 B.C. after the victory against king Mithridates, and was one of Rome's main supporters of Oriental-Hellenistic culture and splendor. His reputation as a magnificent pleasure seeker is all that remains of his rich and versatile nature. For his guests the pleasures began at the start of dinner with the arrival of a large cart brought by a slave, the *sferculum*, upon which sat *patinae*, large platters with tasty and refined foods, and served the *gustatio*, or *promulsi*, our appetizers, of ripened black olives, brine pickled green olives, asparagus, green salad and wine poured into small bowls called *patellae*.

Here is how the 2nd century B.C. poet, Plautus, speaks of the gluttonous parasite of Roman "agape" (meal):

> *I reserve and exercise the ancient and venerable trade of glutton. I nourish it with great care. Of all of my forebears, there was not one of them who did not fill his belly in any other way then by the industriousness of being a parasite. Just like mice, they ravaged everyone else's bread and no one surpassed them in voracity.*

On the tables of the lower echelons of society, cabbage, turnips and other vegetables held their ground. Once, turnips appeared even on the well-to-do tables, after turning them into something more appealing, dyeing them purple and doctoring up the taste by marinating them in mustard.

Here is what Juvenal offers to an invited friend:

> *From the countryside of Tivoli we will have a fat goat, the most tender of the herd, that never fed on grass and never bit any willow, because it has*

more milk than blood. Then there will be mountain asparagus, picked by the farmers when they stop spinning wool, and large eggs still warmed by their hay, with the hen that laid them. In addition, bunches of grapes preserved for many months as they were on the vine, pears from Segni and the Orient. What's more, from the same chest, sweet smelling apples.

Pears, apples, pomegranates and figs were in Italy since very ancient times. Peaches (Persia), apricots (Armenia) and quince (Lebanon) arrived from the provinces of the Empire only during the 1st century A.D., while the lemon, originally from Persia, was introduced later. Grapes and figs were the real champions of fruit on Roman tables. Table grapes, the largest, sweetest and most prized, were gathered not far from the city (suburb), preserved dry or immersed in wine must, cooked wine, or eaten fresh, after being harvested and placed under straw, sawdust or even trellises. Martial describes his friend's greenhouses that used glass and talc to protect the grape shoots this way:

The grape harvest prospers under the protection of a precious transparent substance: your fortunate grape is sheltered and yet is not subtracted from your view. That is how the body of a woman shines through silk; in the same way you can count the pebbles in a transparent lake.

Forty-eight varieties of figs, that is how many the Romans knew of. This bears witness to how much they enjoyed this fruit. They ate figs after the meal as dessert, in combination with something else (*pulmentarium*), or consumed them with bread in substitution for a true meal.

Like other peoples, the Romans acquired a taste for sweets thanks to very ripe fruit, especially figs and above all honey. In Imperial Rome the consumption of "nectar of bees" increased so that it was necessary to import it from the colonies. Prized honey came from Taranto, from Calabria and was imported from Greece. Despite the multiplication of hives, natural honey production was expensive and insufficient to meet the demand. Cheap substitutes appeared: dried fig paste and concentrated grape and date juices were given the name "Phoenician honey". Their production reached such levels that Emperor Diocletian was forced to regulate the sale of authentic and artificial honey.

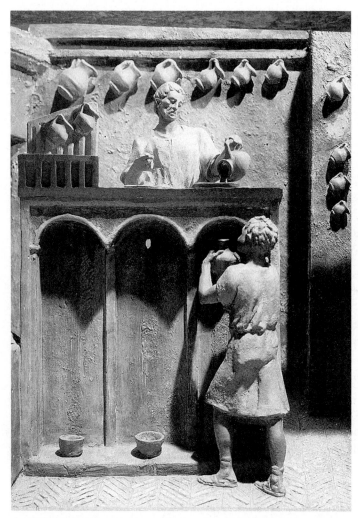

Model of a wine tavern. In the Museum of Roman Civilization, Rome.

For the entire 1st century A.D. the rich consolidated their excessive eating habits: the use of the extremely expensive *laser*, or *Cyrenaic silphium*, increased in an uncontrollable manner, as did its cost, which rose consistently. The use of *laser* became even more in demand in the centuries that followed until its disappearance. The Romans ate the *Partic silphium*, or *asafoetida*, still used today as a spice in Indian cooking. We use garlic instead.

By the beginning of the 2nd century A.D., food consumption was no longer moderate and austerity was no longer in style, to the point where Juvenal wrote:

> *Curius picked the produce from his garden alone and cooked it on his meager fire by himself: a supper disdained even by the most filthy farm laborer, used to savoring tasty sow vulvas in hot inns.*

It seems, as a matter of fact, that sow vulvas and breasts were tasty choices for Roman fine palates, although in time such foods disappeared. Also well liked were boar from Umbria or Lucania, cooked slowly and stuffed; it was for the stuffing that, in an allegoric sense, they called it *Trojan boar.*

And just think that in times gone by, meat remained an exceptional food. Livestock animals for butchering were introduced at the beginning of the 3rd century B.C. to supply the ever growing demand of developing urban life. Pigs were courtyard animals and unrivaled donors of meat dishes. According to Varro, nature donated the pig for feasting. Even Pliny gave honors to the pig:

> *No animal furnishes more food to gluttony than the pig, given that its meat has about fifty different tastes, while that of the others have but one.*

Once washed thoroughly and wrapped in cloth, meat was preserved in cool, dark and well ventilated places for a short period; or in the cold, taking advantage of the snow in the hinterland regions. Drying, smoking and salting was instead used whenever it was necessary to preserve it for long periods.

Roman cooking was also rich in fish and oysters, the latter were served with *panis ostrearius*, hunks of crunchy bread. Shellfish was generally well liked. Here are the rules set by Horace:

> *The slimy seashells fill up when there is a full moon, but not all seas produce good ones: better than the murex of Baia is the Lucrino clam, the oysters from Circeo or the urchins from Miseno are excellent, the refined Taranto boasts easy to open scallops.*

Plautus leads off a hymn to Roman fishermen that describes their lowly existence:

Our clothing tells you how rich we are: here are the hooks and the poles, light gear that keeps us alive; we try to fish for marine oysters, clams, sea urchins, striated pinnae and balani and shellfish; and then we go fishing with hooks among the rocks. Our nourishment comes from the sea, but if nothing else, weariness overcomes us and not even one fish is hauled in, in that case we return wet and salty, and we go hiding to bed without supper. And when the sea is rough, like now, we have no other hope but to gather some seashells washed up on the beach.

Because of their habit of seasoning with flavorful sauces, such as *garum*, all Roman dishes were very tasty. *Garum* was a widely used condiment in antiquity, made by placing fish and guts from several kinds of fish under salt with various spices. Other types of sauces were also used. These were based on oil, spices, wine, vinegar, and black pepper. Vinegar was not only made from wine, left to acidify with added fruits, herbs or roots, but also dates, figs, fermented with lemon juice and toasted barley.

The quest for culinary delight reached such high proportions of gluttony in ancient Rome that phrases were coined. The throat hurts more than the sword *(plus gula, quam gladius)*, stated Cicero; while Seneca said that:

The Romans eat to vomit and vomit to eat.

Horace declared:

The overloaded body with food weighs down the spirit and bears to Earth the divine breath that animates us.

After the rich feasts, guests were bad off because they ate so much and especially because of the amount of food processing that went into cooking some dishes. During Augustus' reign, the famous physician Celsus attempted to establish a cure to after-meal problems by dividing the foods according to nutritional value: for Celsus, rich foods were grains and cereals, poor foods were cabbage, and fruit with pulp. The Emperor Claudius ate ten melons to wet his appetite; to strengthen his voice, the divine Nero chewed leeks. And Augustus? He was able to stand drinking no more than five and a half liters of wine without vomiting. At least that is what Suetonius said.

Rich feasts were dominated by people bathed in gold and fat; especially those organized by the miserable new class of rich servants who had become landholders. Thus, Petronius referred to Trimalcione and all the corruption that had by now invaded Rome.

As Nero's mentor, Seneca could well say:

Money falls on certain people as in a sewer.

In *De Re Coquinaria*, a cookbook attributed to Marcus Gavius Apicius, there is an ever growing custom of using various sauces to prepare every kind of dish, and there is a description of the continuous attempt to render such dishes more and more elaborate in taste. The author is with great likelihood Apicius who perhaps lived during the reign of Tiberius, between the 1st century B.C. and 1st century A.D. and who even undertook a long sea voyage just to fish for large Libyan shrimp. This was the same Apicius who committed suicide because the 10 million sesterzii in his possession would not allow him to continue his lifestyle. Seneca commented on that gesture quite ironically.

The mortal drink must have been the healthiest thing that Apicius ever drank in his life.

Be that as it may, the recipes and instructions contained in the book influenced gastronomy until the Middle Ages.

The aforementioned delicacies regarded wealthy tables and were certainly out of a poor man's reach. The latter continued to live on a meager diet, based mostly on barley bread and olives. Often the drinks such as wine, apple juice and others, were taken with olives that tasted of prolonged pickling in brine.

Olive oil for Roman cooking was considered a precious dressing that the upper-brachet loved to use to flavor all dishes. Highly prized oil was the *onfacinum* or *oleum viride* made from tart green olives (such as those produced in Venafro). This was a clear and odorless oil used both for cooking and as a balm for body care. It was the best quality they had and that reflected in the high price. *Oleum maturum* or *commune* was used by the plebeians and came from ripe black olives. It was less prized and above all very inexpensive. The oil given to slaves, instead, was the poorest quality, worse for taste and color. That oil, given the name *cibarium oleum*, came from soft olives found on the ground. Before the olive culture spread, they probably used animal fat, principally pork fat. This is also because butter as a condiment was unknown.

In the different epochs, however, Roman kitchens were always stocked with fish, olives, wild game, garden produce such as lettuce, leeks, common mallow, broad beans, cabbage, chard, onions, fruit in season, prunes, grapes, pears, practically everything that their land could grow. It is worth noting, for instance, that Pompeii was renowned for its figs and cabbage as well as broad beans and onions, from which a very tasty seasoning was made. Today, after nineteen centuries, a pan containing the remains of this condiment has been brought to light from the ruins of the once splendid city.

Top left, next page. *Portable stove in terracotta. In the National Archeology Museum, Naples.*

Middle. *Terracotta crock pot on a three-legged iron stand. In the National Archeology Museum, Naples.*

Top right. *A mosaic in the atrium of the House of Umbricius Scaurus: an amphora for garum with the name of the producer. Pompeii.*

Bottom right. *A mosaic with fish, a moray, an octopus, a large lobster in the center. Origin unknown. In the British Museum, London.*

Bottom left. *A detailed floor mosaic depicting the remains of food from a feast. In the Gregorian Museum, Vatican City.*

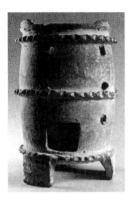

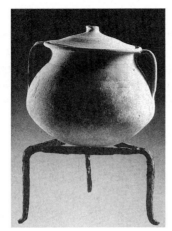

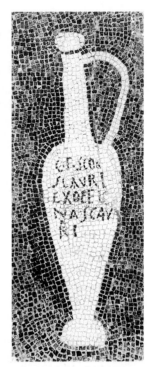

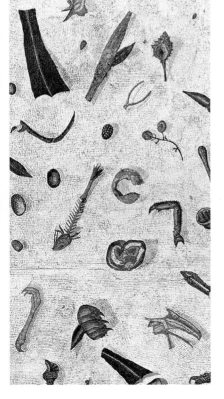

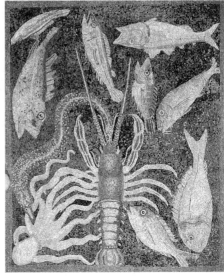

In ancient times, the Romans had such little use for wine that they did not allow their young to drink it and prohibited it to women. The drinking was reserved particularly for worshipping their gods. Then this custom was abolished, including the *ius osculi*, that allowed a husband to determine with a kiss whether or not his wife disobeyed this order. Contact with the Etruscans first, and then with the Greek colonies in southern Italy led to the expansion in wine use. Although limited and poor quality, Roman wine making is documented already in the 5th century B.C., but continued for a long time with unrefined methods, and scarce results. Pliny narrates that Cinea, the ambassador sent by Pyrrhus to Rome in 279 B.C. to negotiate peace, mocked the vinegar tasting wine made on the Albani hills.

During the period that marked the maximum expansion of the wine culture, from the 2nd century B.C. onward, there were almost 200 varieties of grapevine, even if Pliny estimated that only eighty were worthy of mention. The celebrated Falernian wine was also called blaze, perhaps because it was so strong that it burned itself up aging and ended up being set on fire. Massicum, Cecubum (both made in the renowned *ager falernum*), Albanum, Sabinum, the wines from Sorrento and those from Sezze were equally renowned. Even the wine from Verona, *noble vinegar* in the words of Tiberius, and *vinum pucinum* from Aquileia, that permitted the empress Livia to reach the venerable age of 86 years, were esteemed. Famous too were the vineyards in Capua and the wine from Vesuvius, called Vesbius by Martial, the wine from Messina (*vinum mamertinum*) and the wine from Syracuse. Wine from the Vatican hills is remembered for its scarce quality that caused it to be used to cut the noble Falernum. A certain Tucca could not escape the Martial satire for having attempted to poison Falernum with that awful wine.

> It is a crime to poison Falernum: your guests perhaps deserved to be put to death, but such an important amphora did not.

Beer was considered a crude drink, fit only for provincials, barbarians and for the general poor. Gallic beer (*cervesia*) held some amount of credit, but also Iberic beer (*Hispania* beer) became known, especially after a procedure was found to guarantee freshness over a long time.

The Romans loved sweets: confections and sweets were in great demand and ever present at the end of large feasts. Sweets were highly refined. The great chefs indulged their whims by bringing to the table thrushes made from rye, shellfish made from quince apples and other delicious dishes (Trimalcione's dinner). But there were also seedless dates, stuffed with walnuts and pine nuts then fried in honey, *mustacei*, cakes dipped in wine must and needed with cheese and baked in the oven on bay leaves, and *globi* which resembled today's Neapolitan *struffoli*. Finally, there was the forefather of the Sicilian *cassata*, which can be seen in a wall painting from Poppaea's villa at Oplontis, just walking distance from Pompeii.

There is no doubt, as can be gathered by watching how the cuisine evolved over the centuries, that Apicius' cooking, the cooking so full of *garum*, had a long domination in antiquity. It even appears that many recipes, although modified in different epochs, reached renaissance kitchens; a sign of the high degree of refinement and value in taste achieved by ancient Roman cuisine.

Coena with Lucullus

Appetizers: Hard boiled eggs, sea urchins from Capo Miseno, clams from Taranto, tuna from Calcedonia, oysters from Lucrino, ham from Gaul, fried snails with Cuma onions, olives, Falernian wine after clarification with pigeon eggs.

Courses: Sturgeon from Rhodes, morays from Bacoli in wine from Chios, peacock stuffed with sausage and Puteolan *ofelle*, roast pig stuffed with fig-eaters, roast chicken with salad, rabbit shoulder, goose liver pate, fried *scari* from Miseno and shrimp from Formia.

Dessert: Hazel nuts from Nola, almonds from Agrigento, raisins from Sicily, dates from Egypt, fruit from the Phlegrean Fields (*annurche* apples, yellow peaches, watermelon, melons), pastries, honey sweetened wines.

Garum

Garum was the famous fish sauce used by the ancients to flavor just about everything: vegetables, meat and even fruit. Although this practice may appear to be very distant from our taste, it must have been highly valued and held worthy of the maximum culinary respect to appear in so many recipes. Apicius, a person dedicated to the culinary arts whose writings have reached us, placed a sprinkle of garum in almost every dish. Such a vast expansion of garum should not escape the many writers, politicians, philosophers and playwrights who find the pabulum to feed their ideas in everyday things. Pliny the Elder honored this "rot of putrefying things" obtained by fermenting fish guts under salt, probably the most common, the most accessible and therefore the most widespread.

The quality of some different kinds of garum became so high and the costs so prohibitive, at least for most consumers, that Cato attacked it as an extravagance on the level of cosmetics and perfumes. Seneca, Martial and Pliny the Elder agreed with Cato in this final word, underscoring, however, the high quality and refinement of the product, skillfully prepared and with a unique taste, color of honeyed wine, good enough, according to Pliny, to drink. He had, of course, to have been speaking of the best garum, that made with the blood of still throbbing mackerel, even if the less renowned and costly product must have been the garum made with sea bass and anchovies. Garum, true gluttony for every palate, withstood the fall of the Roman Empire: a thousand years after the tragedy of Pompeii, the Byzantine Empire continued to be crazy about garum.

The garum trade flourished in the Mediterranean basin. From the production areas in the coastal cities of *Campania Felix* (Pompeii), Gaul (Antibes) and southern Spain, garum reached affluent households as a distinctive product, sealed in small amphoras upon which tags were attached that revealed the origin and producer. A small amphora uncovered in Pompeii held the inscription *garum sociorum,* a product made with the finest fish in numerous plants throughout Spain, favored by the bountifulness in raw materials, mackerel that literally slipped into fishermen's nets during migration, and the numerous salt mines.

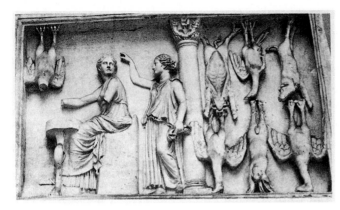

Relief showing a chicken, rabbit and small pig vender. In the Torlonia Museum, Rome.

This happy combination, among plenty of fish, wealth in salt and a specialized labor force made many entrepreneurs rich. One of them, A. Umbricius Scaurus, even had a splendid tomb erected in *Via dei Sepolcri*, Pompeii. In his elegant house, a floor mosaic repeats the image of a single handled anphora in every corner, the kind they used locally, upon which the product name can be read (*gari flos scombri* – the flower of mackerel garum) and the name of the producer. Pompeii exported large quantities of it, mostly garum of Scaurus made with tuna, morays, and mackerel. They sealed it in flasks packed in straw and shipped it along sea routes to the whole Roman world. The salt needed was supplied by the numerous salt deposits in the city. The Herculean door, in fact, was called the salt door and the garum was prepared here in large vats that must have let escape a strange, even acrid odor.

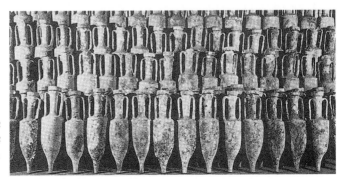

Wine amphoras from the Imperial age. In the Naval Museum, Albenga.

Actually, garum was made by fermenting fish under salt; a rather concentrated salt bath, enough so to float an egg. The sauce must have been more or less liquid with a color that changed according to the type of fish used and spices added. The thinnest part, with less culinary and economic value, was obtained after straining several times. This fraction was called *liquamen*, a macabre sounding name, but always largely used in reference to food. The dregs, called *alec* or *allex*, were used in medicine to heal wounds.

Garum, black pepper, wine and oil, were the main ingredients of all fish sauces. Starting with them, one could invent the most varied kinds of sauces for the most refined and hard-to-please palates. Always, according to Apicius, the ideal sauce to flavor grilled mullet had to be prepared by heating vinegar, wine, garum and oil, to which one had to add black pepper, rue, *levisticum* (privet) and pine nuts all finely chopped, and then honey. Tuna seemed to be particularly appetizing when basted with a sauce made by mixing black pepper, *levisticum*, celery seed, mint, rue, dates and honey melted in wine, vinegar and oil. The quince apples took the place of dates when the fish was a sea bream, while Damascus prunes were a delicacy for the moray eels.

The art of bread making

The Romans enjoyed hot and fragrant bread to go along with a little cheese, an onion grown in the suburb gardens or better yet with a cup of wine drunk at the bar of an inn.

A lot of water had passed under the bridge since spelt flour, cooked in salt and water, was their dietary staple. That was the famous *puls*, that they tried to render more palatable by mixing with broad beans (*puls fabata*). It was very difficult for some to agree with Cato the Elder who seemed to hold something against bread's wide distribution since its large scale introduction to the cuisine in the 2nd century B.C. It was good to try and reintroduce more sober-minded uses and customs and return to the good old days, but why deprive the people of bread made with husked durum wheat-germ flour to return to *puls* and spelt *focaccia* bread. Agreed that for about three centuries spelt was very important in the economic and social history of Rome. There is no doubt that like the Greek barley *maza*, Roman *focaccia* bread, garnished with cheese, olives, eggs, mushrooms, meat or everything imaginable, continued to be the main dish of the Romans. But why hold it against bread?

It did not set well with the baker that someone could speak badly of bread, also because bread sales were his greatest income. The name by which bread was known (*pistor*) came from the ancient word for servants (*pistores*) who ground the grains of spelt

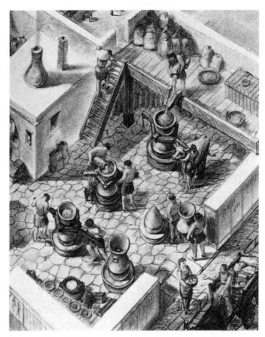

Scene of grinding and storing grain in a pistrinum at Pompeii.

in mortars after a quick toasting over the fire to block fermentation. In conclusion, we need to ask what Cato could have known about all the kinds of bread that differ in shape, size, oven times and uses?

The baker was a fortunate man; not to mention rich. Unlike others, he could boast a unique specialization in pastries, those *pistores dulciarii* that were so in style. The baker, though, had a hard job. He had to get up early in the morning to purchase wheat supplements during festivals, games and other occurrences that drew in people to feed.

Wheat was ground in a mill attached to the house or, in the case of the baker Modestus from Pompeii, in the *tablinum* and in the garden of the house rearranged for such a purpose. The donkey and slave alternated in turning the grindstone by pushing wooden poles stuck into square holes on the upper, moveable part of the grinding wheel. Once the wheat was turned into flour, it fell to the round base, ready to undergo other fruitful changes. Making bread dough required tremendous patience: just the right amount of yeast, water, salt, all mixed in the large circular tubs by animal power. After having risen, the bread was shaped into round loaves, like sweet bread, divided into eight pieces to make it easier to eat. The loaves were all the same size and weight, as the contractor ordered. The proud baker signed his work. He stamped it above the factory brand. This is what Proculus, the prince of bakers, did in Pompeii. Loaves were placed in the oven previously cleaned of ash by dry sorghum stalk brooms.

Brick ovens cooked normal bread made from chickpeas or rye; noble ovens made from terracotta shingles baked wheat bread. Gentlemen preferred *mundus* bread displayed on the sales counter.

Of course, the farmer who lived far from the city could not reap the benefits from progress in bread making arts. He had to make do with his own, like Similus, the uncouth farmer described by Virgil.

Having finished the work of grinding, with hands filled with flour he sifts and shakes it: the bran remains stuck in the holes above while the true pure flour rains down, then it gets toasted and piled up on a smooth table. He pours warm water over it and kneads water and flour. The dough gets hard, he bends it sidewise and the loaves dry; a pinch of salt on top.

The astute baker sold bread from door to door when business was slow. A young man with just the right voice for the occasion loaded a portable oven on his back and moved to a busy place, usually the forum, and attracted the passersby with songs of praise to biscuits.

Nineteen centuries after the catastrophe that befell Pompeii, the 81 loaves in Modestus' oven came to light by removing the small oven door, silent and now cold witnesses of a far too long oven time.

Quick and youthful snacks

In southern Mediterranean cities, the street is still everyone's home, refuge, and meeting point, but also stage upon which everyday life is carried out. The numerous boutiques that lined the busily traveled streets of Roman cities attracted strollers. By selling warm food and beverages, the eateries and taverns represented an important moment in the day for refreshment and chit-chat.

The most frequented establishment in antiquity, still recognizable today by its structure, was the *thermopolium*, an ancient snack-bar. Here, food was eaten while standing around large brick counters along one side of the room opened to the street with one or two other sides forming a right angle. Huge terracotta urns with wide mouths and even wider necks were fixed in place and covered with multicolored marble. When the terracotta lids were removed the air filled with the smells from their contents: food and perhaps beverages that caused customers to elbow each other to get in close, especially during frequent festivals.

The proprietor would stick a long wooden spoon through the wide open mouth to remove dried or smoked food, legumes, vegetables and the delicious olives that tasted of long brine pickling and that went so well with drink: wine mixed with water and honey, myrrh, or apple juice. The connoisseurs asked for *posca*, a divine tasting drink made from water, beaten eggs and vinegar. This was drunk from beautiful cups that decorated the wooden or marble shelves along the wall or counter. For those who preferred hot and steaming food, there was a small terracotta or metal stove resting on the floor or on the inside end of the counter. Sometimes there was an oven in the adjoining room. These were used to bake sweet smelling *focaccia* bread, hot juicy cakes, and watery legume stews that made mouths water.

Patrons who wanted to get away from the crowd and eat a full course meal while seated at a table, or spend the night to give the pack animals a rest, asked for hospitality at the numerous taverns *(tabernae/cauponae)* that offered a watery broad bean or cabbage soup, wonderful smelling and flavorful mashed Indian pepper and Nocerin garlic together with a cup of domestic wine. There was something for everyone's taste and budget, vegetable and legume dishes, especially chickpeas, eggs and various cheeses, roasted meats and sausage, even wild game such as fish, shellfish, truffles and mushrooms. For those with assets and a desire to spend them on drink, there was Falernian wine to be had in the long amphora that the proprietor tapped for such occasions; paying attention not to pour resin from the seal into the

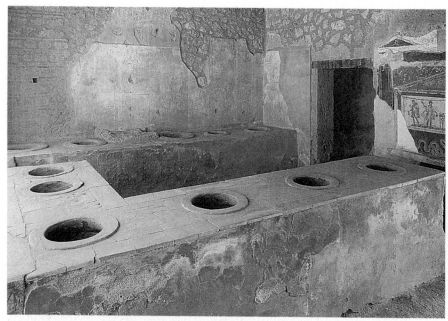

Thermopolium on Via dell'Abbondanza. Pompeii.

Bottom left. *Emblem of the Tor Marancia villa showing stores of dates, asparagus, fish and chicken. Half of the 2nd century A.D. In the Vatican Museums, Vatican City.*

Lararium from the kitchen in the Casa del Maiale (House of the Pig). Pompeii.

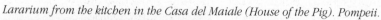

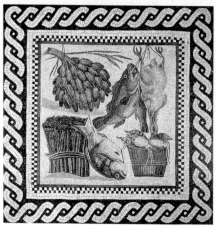

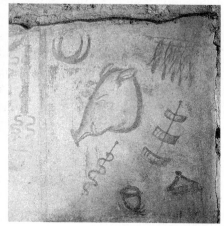

lucky cups. The salamis and cheeses hanging from the rafters of the room must have been a delight to see, the wine amphoras leaning against the wall were an invitation to sweet company.

Those who went to establishments in the capital, especially those catering to commoners, were reminded of scenes that would not make one want to dine there. They were dirty, smoky and greasy, poorly furnished, with few rickety tables, chairs and stools teaming with tiny summer bugs. The habit of purchasing precooked meals to be eaten at home, or buying just hot water and coals to cook the few available foods, was dictated by the lack of a simple stove.

It is known that the innkeeper's wife had the well being of her guests in mind, especially those well off; so she provided them with pleasures of the flesh, not only the edible kind, but those up in the cubicles on the floor above, or a great variety of games, some gambling, to facilitate wine consumption and make the *copa* even happier.

Virgil described just how the innkeeper's wife Sira attracted wayfarers.

Sira the innkeeper's wife wears a Greek style turban and sways to the music of castanets. She dances unrestrained and enraptured in the smoke filled room. The provocative dance accompanies the sharp rhythmic beats of wooden drum sticks... What's more, dried in the "fiscelle" we have persimmons, and yellow plums, and blood red black berries, cone-shaped bunches of beautiful grapes and green watermelon, and ruby apples and chestnuts. Bread, wine, love, all share this house freely with gaiety. Hey servant, bring this to the table, it is time, uncut wine and dice! And he who thinks about afterwards, leaves early in a bad mood! Death is on our heels, and we recite this warning in silent syllables: Here I am, I'm coming, oh men. Enjoy yourselves.

These establishments were used as houses of ill repute. They drank, ate, and gambled in the main hall of the tavern on the ground floor off the street. On the next floor, or out in the garden, one or two rooms allowed clients to meet the innkeeper's wife or the waitress for a brief moment of pleasure. Unsurprisingly, there was a phallic symbol at the entranceway to protect everyone from the evil eye, but also indicated the nature of the establishment, without shame. A traveler from Isernia told of an inscription erected on the innkeepers' tomb from his town, L. Calindius Eroticus and his wife Fannia Voluptas:

> *"Innkeeper, let's settle the bill".*
> *"You had a sextarius (equal to 0.54 liter) of wine, for the wine: one as (Roman coin). For the stew, two asses".*
> *"Agreed".*
> *"For the girl, eight asses".*
> *"All right".*
> *"Hay for the mule, two asses".*
> *"That mule will be my ruin".*

Even Horace experimented with the duality of the inns, to his great displeasure. One day he had to stop in a miserable inn somewhere near Benevento. The hall was full of smoke and lousy food. Worse yet, he waited all night long in vane for the servant girl who promised him that she would visit his room.

A landlord from Pompeii named Asellina had three servant girls working for her, Egle the Greek, and Zmirina and Maria from the near East, to distract her clients. The blacksmith who forged the metal boiling pot in Asellina's inn was a master in the art of sealing containers: in her tavern located on *Via dell'Abbondanza* it challenged the eruption and the long nights. Found in the heart of the excavations, the pot was still filled with century old water.

A feast in Pompeii

The gastronomic scene of the Roman world changed with time as a consequence of trade, near and distant wars, and fashion. Cato's unrefined meal, made up largely of cereals and vegetables flavored with simple condiments, salt, oil, vinegar and fragrant spices from the Roman countryside, seemed to succumb to the extravagance of the rich who ate precious fowl, peacock, dormice and snails, in a display of questionable culinary refinement. Cabbage and turnips were ever present on the table of the common folk, but lost their once held appeal, when besieged by new tastes.

What happened to Cato's rules that described the responsibilities of the housewife?

You, peasant, must make sure the housewife does her chores – takes care to cook food for you and for the country family. That she has many hens and eggs: dried pears, apples, figs, raisins, sorb apples in cooked grape must, and pears and grapes in jars and in buried pots: and Scanziane apples in terracotta pots and others that are usually preserved, even the wild game. Let her devote herself to putting up all these supplies every year. She had also better know how to make good flour and fine spelt.

The ancient health virtue of the cabbage described by Cato the Elder 200 years before Christ seems to have been forgotten:

Eaten raw in vinegar, cooked in oil or grease, cabbage drives out and cures all. When struck down without strength, with rue grass it fights fever. If at a feast you want to drink hard and eat heartily, eat five leaves of cabbage: you will retain the appearance of one who has neither drunk, nor eaten and you can continue to drink as much as you like.

Bearing witness to this long vegetarian period in their history are names and surnames of many Roman families. The Fabii's, who took their name from *faba* (broad beans) farmed by their forefathers. There was Licinius Stolone, so named from the strawberry *stolon*, and Lentuli's from lentils. From the Valeria people there was the Lactucini branch who clearly derived from lettuce (*lactuca*). And what is to say of the famous Cicero whose name derived from *cicer*, the miserly chickpea, inspired by the large mole on his face? The Romans were reneging the title of "grass eaters," so dear to Plautus.

According to a project made by Vitruvius, the famous Roman architect, the length of the dining room of this wealthy Pompeian was twice as long as the width. Reclining couches were set up on three sides of the *mensa*, that low wide and square table where platters were set, to leave one side free for serving. There could be three at the table, a perfect number for the size of the couches. The fashion of eating like the Greeks, comfortably reclining on the left elbow, with the head held at the height of the table, between pillows, had made its debut into wealthy circles.

*Burned foods from Pompeii. In the
National Archeology Museum, Naples.*

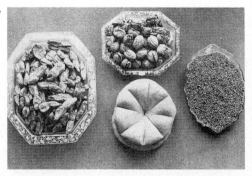

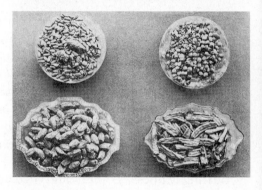

Pillows functioned as a partition between guests. According to the best tradition, slaves would rush to wash and dry the feet of the table companions, and extend a linen cloth on the pillows. The host's toes would smell of fresh water and perfume poured from a pitcher. This issue completed, everything would be ready, even the personal napkins (*mappae*) that the guests opened on the tablecloth to later fill with tasty left over morsels, hoping to continue the rite in their abodes.

But what of the woman of the household who wanted to participate in the feast. Immediately a servant would bring a stool (*subsellum*) and set it near the place taken up by the husband on the couch, because it was inconvenient for women to eat half reclining. The *pocillatores* opened the wine amphoras. These were labelled with the name of the vineyard and year. Using a strainer the *pocillatores* carefully avoided contaminating the wine with pitch and resin needed to preserve it. They poured it into craters already two-thirds filled with clean water.

Wine from *Setia* was an excellent aperitif, but some appetizers served required aged *mulsum* cut with honey. The name itself given to appetizers (*gustus* or *pomulsis*) testifies this union. Leaves from mint, mallow, corn rocket, green and black olives bathed in vinegar, pig breast flavored with tuna fish garum, fresh water crabs and shrimp were all common appetizers.

The cooks (*stuctores*) prepared many courses, all different and with assured breathtaking effect: peacock eggs with fig-eater dipped in egg yokes with long peppercorns, the allspice derived from drying the pods before they ripen, kidneys and African figs, gray mullet and lobster, and finally the roasts. What a delight for eyes and palate! A chicken stuffed with goose and still virgin pig liver surrounded by small boars, almost to suggest a purifying sucking. The servants carried out platters, washed and dried hands that worked as skillful as forks, filled wine cups. They did so with moderation because uninhibited drinking began later. But be that as it may, the generous wines would soon take the place of the no langer suitable *mulsum*.

The third course (*secundae mensae*) would be fresh and dried fruit, even dates and pistachio nuts, pastries and sweet edibles, served on elegant silver trays. Everyone would have been awaiting the *commissatio*. The election of the feast king (*rex convivii*) was quick and the most illustrious guest of the evening would hold the job of *arbiter bibendi*. Clearing the table of plates and leftovers, the king would take on the role and order the servants to bring stronger bodied wine worthy of such a table, boasting of the host's rich cellars: the *cecubum* and *falernum*. The amphora carried the labels (*lituli*) with the denomination of the wine, the kind and the year it was made. The cups would pass, luckily not filled to the brim because the far-sighted king would like the evening to be happy, but above all long.

There was entertainment: acrobats passed through blazing rings, musicians played double flute or the *sambuca* and dancers danced. A clown, in reality a grotesque midget with the deformed nose, molested the delighted ballerinas. It is said that in Rome the dancers from Gades, the current Cadiz, were highly praised for their castanets and obscene shouts that set the beat for swinging hips that aroused eroticism in the guests.

With their heads crowned with flowers, and by now with no stock-
ings, the table companions would talk loudly and drink until late, passing the summer night in a flood of talk. Strengthened by an edict from
Claudius and advice from physicians, the table companions would gave
themselves up to different noises, all healthy: the belch was the *"last
word of wisdom"*.

Unlike the Greeks, the Romans let their feasts get out of control.
They exceeded the ritual of pleasure and voluptuousness in every way.
It was a world of illusion and disguise. At Roman feasts the number
one thing was food, transformed with great culinary and gastronomic
skill, to give dishes the appearance of what they weren't. Eat, drink and
get sick: the traditional impression of the Roman orgy, a certain impression of imperial Rome, where everything was out of proportion, just as
Rome itself and its inhabitants.

The epitaph decided upon by the figure who emerged from Petronius' witty pen, Trimalcione, for his tomb is emblematic:

> *Here rests Gaius Pompeius Trimalcione Mecenatianus. He was decreed
> the seviratus during his absence. He could have been in all the ducuries
> of Rome, but had no want. Pious, strong and faithful, he rose from noth-
> ing, left thirty million sesterzii, and never once listened to a philosopher.*

Christian agape

The Pedagogue is an etiquette book written by Clement Alexandrine
in the 2nd century A.D. Among the other things that it mentions, one
can read these rules intended for a simple diet:

> *If others live to eat, we eat to live. Thus, nutrition must be simple, never
> refined, easy to eat and soothe digestion, to avoid any illness and to
> maintain one healthy and moderate.*

The Pedagogue also recommended which foods to favor: bread,
mostly roasted fish, onions, olives, legumes, milk and cheese, cooked
beverages, and avoid sauces.

Early Christian meals were not a whole lot different than their counterparts. They offered greater frugality, together with the choice of simpler and inexpensive foods. Unlike the excesses of imperial Roman cuisine and some customs then in use, often reinforced by the advice of doctors and even by imperial edicts, the Christians were obedient to the rules laid down by The Pedagogue. They avoided making noise at the

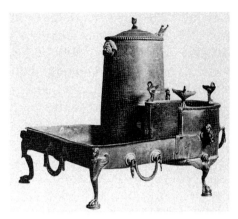

Bronze boiler used to create steam. In the National Archeology Museum, Naples.

table, were careful not to get dirty, did not speak with their mouths full, and waited patiently their turn for food to be passed around. There is a great deal of good sense in these manners.

One could drink wine, but not overdo it. St. Paul recommended wine as a medicine. St. John Crisostomo and St. Basil Magnus (4th century) agreed that wine was a gift of God and as such must be used in moderation and sparingly. For the *Aquarii*, true censures of customs and extremists, wine was the work of the devil and must be strongly prohibited. In memory of the long wine making tradition passed down from the Greeks and Romans, wine was cut with water, likely in the same proportions in use (one third wine, two thirds water).

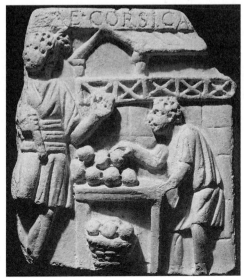

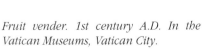

Fruit vender. 1st century A.D. In the Vatican Museums, Vatican City.

Funeral dinners took on great importance for the Christians, revived from the pagan Roman world. They became an integral part of the devotion toward the dead. During these feasts, all forms of sadness were set aside to celebrate the future happiness of the deceased in his spiritual lifting. Such feasts, indeed, were called *refrigeria*, or receptions for the body and spirit and took place at the grave, even over it, on boards set up as needed. This can be seen on portrayals in early Christian catacombs. The boards on which they ate were stationary or mobile, set up for the occasion on the anniversary of the death of a loved one – the *dies natalis.* The meal (*agape*), at least in the beginning, was frugal, with bread and fish, somewhat like the daily meal, accompanied by wine heated in amphoras or terracotta pots placed on food warmers. In the course of time, participation at such feasts even took on a role of public charity towards the more needy.

Everyday life was scarcely portrayed in these scenes of feasting, being that they were above all a way to depict biblical scenes and symbolically the spirituality of the deceased, with the exception made for scenes depicting trades or portraits.

On the level of nutritional value, Christianity is the direct heir of the Roman world and its traditions: bread, wine and oil, the ideal summary of the Mediterranean dietary model, are also products that the Christian liturgy has rendered sacred, the indispensable tools of the trade for the champions and broadcasters of the new faith. Indeed, in the hagiographic accounts of the high Middle Ages, bishops and abbots were intent on seeding cereal and planting grapevines around the churches and newly founded monasteries.

7 Grapevines

A gift from Dionysus

Wine is a gift from Dionysus. The fertile grapevine that produces it needs to be cared for, trained in its growth, pruned, and cherished. Wine cannot be drunk without precautions. Dionysus alone drinks wine straight and natural, without any risk. But men must obey a series of rules that define the good use of wine, a series of steps dictated by the god. Last in a line of Olympian gods, Dionysus was beloved by mortals. He was present in their everyday affairs, on the sides of craters, on the bottom of cups, anywhere images appear that evoke the *comos* (parade of drinkers) or the symposium.

This is how Euripides, in the Bacchanti, delivered the eulogy of wine and Dionysus:

> *This new god, that you mock, I wouldn't know how great he will be in Hellas, tomorrow. Young men, there are two fundamental things for humans: the goddess Demeter, that is to say, the earth, however you wish to call her, because she nurtures mortals with cereal, and he who comes after, his emulation, the son of Semele (Dionysus), who spread grape juice among men, which offers respite to the bread of mortals, when they drink the liquor of the vine and give themselves up to sleep, oblivious of the daily hustle, for which there is no other remedy.*

Women could pour wine, under the protection of Dionysus (drinking it was forbidden). Drinking it straight was unusual, wine was seen as a poison that drives one mad. One needed to dominate wine, water it down, according to ancient canons and passed down over the years, the amounts had to be just right. The proportion of the mixture defined the moderation of the drinker or his intemperance.

Despite the distribution of grapevines throughout Greece, not much care was given to them. The most prized vineyards, those that produced the famous *Taso* or *Chios* wines, likely received more attention than others. If one is to believe an inscription from the 3rd century B.C. Rhodes, prized vineyards had to be flat, cereals and legumes cultivated between the rows parallel to the grapes, while fig and almond trees could grow haphazardly throughout the vineyard.

In such a varied landscape as that found in Greece, the climatic conditions and the soil must have influenced the choice of support for the vine shoots and the height that the strains could reach. Climbing vines or low vines grew on the windy islands. Grapevines did well on trellises, on yokes protected by walls or on crossed arbors and trees.

Wine developed into the main beverage of the Greeks. From Thrace, Taso and Chios, it was exported into Athens and other cities that requested it in terracotta amphoras, with very good seals to assure excellent aging. Greek wines, especially the reds, must have been strong, with a greater than 15 proof alcohol content, 18 proof for the wine from Taso. It is no wonder then that they cut it with water, or mixed it with weaker wines. Strong wines underwent slow fermentation and long aging.

The customary magniloquence of the Greeks can also be found in the descriptions of wine. The red wine, tending towards black, was compared to purple or to blood, while white wine had a yellowish color. There were tart wines or dry, sweet and lovable, light or strong. There were warm wines that gave one strength, or those without vigor. All these terms were used to describe the quality of wine and seem to bear witness to the custom of drinking somewhat valuable wines, at least in the classes that were better off socially. The peasant farmer got along with a pleasant light wine made from the dregs of seeds and skins, even vinegar. He had a sad life, but made a profit selling grapes and grape must from which dark and strong wine was made, full of flavor after aging. This was the crop so sought after and paid dearly for on the table of the rich.

Local white wines were of modest quality and did not travel well. Some white wines were presented at the table of the wealthy who had a taste for strong wine. Such a beverage was made from sun ripened raisins. Sometimes they added cooked must, a precursor of the Roman *defrutum*, to render it even sweeter and stronger. This system not only made the buyers happy, but guaranteed preservation on long sea voyages. Even Galen remembers these characteristics:

> *The best suited wine against fever is watery; it is a white wine of fluid make-up and does not have any of the qualities that characterize other wines. It is neither dry, nor bitter, sweet or acid, it has no smell. But it is for this that it is unique among wines and is able to ward off the harmful effects of water and those of wine. Every nation has some wine of this sort. In Italy there is the weak Sabinum that is given to someone with a fever... but abroad they ignore them, and for two reasons, because they are produced everywhere and in modest amounts and because they do not travel well on long sea voyages, the reason why traders cannot export it to other countries.*

Despite the hard life, the wine-maker must not have had it so bad, when not called to arms to defend his sacred boarders. Aristophanes places these words in the mouth of the wine-maker Trigeus:

> *I take no pleasure in fighting, but to stay near the fire and drink with dear friends, burning the dry tinder in summer, and roasting chickpeas and placing acorns over the fire, and meanwhile smooching with the servant girl while my wife bathes... Up with you wife, roast three measures of beans and mix them with grain, and take out the dried figs.*

Wine-making was very different from today: fermentation in tubs was not universal and, in any case, it was never left long enough. This made preserving wine rather difficult. One widely used technique was to mix the wine with salty water or other ingredients, probably with a system currently used in Greece to make resin wine, although literary sources give no information on the addition of resin in classical times. To give wine a spicy aroma, thyme, mint, cinnamon or honey were added. Barley flour and cheese turned wine into an aphrodisiac, at

least this is what the Nestor cup made in Rhodes and found at Lacco
Ameno, on the isle of Ischia, declares:

> *Whomever drinks of this cup will immediately be filled with the desire of
> the beautifully crowned Aphrodite.*

Wine made for immediate use was placed in goatskin or pigskin
sacks. Wine for export was poured into large terracotta containers, the
famous *pithoi* that could hold hundreds of liters, and then in clay amphoras lined inside with pitch. The handles of the amphoras were
marked with the name of the merchant or wine-maker or certain local
magistrates, to guarantee quality. The famous wines, such as those from
Taso, were protected by trade laws that condemned fraud.

Long live the grapevine

> *The earth gives many fruits and the inhabitants, taking care in cultivat-
> ing it, are able to make it bountiful with fruit and not only to sustain
> themselves...The fields are made up of vast plains separated by many
> well-farmed hills...*

This is how Diodorus Siculus described the fertile land of Etruria
when drawing from older sources at the end of the 2nd century B.C.
The grapevine was introduced to Italy by the Greek colonies: the same
derivation of the word *vinum*, both in Etruscan and Latin, is from the
Greek word *oinos*. Not everyone is convinced of this interpretation. The
organized growing of *vitis silvestris* perhaps comes from the 7th century
B.C., as the numerous Etruscan wine amphoras found in tombs seem to
bear out. The word *vinum* derives from the Latin *vitis*, demonstrating
contact with the prior Latin culture that had no written language.

However things may have gone, the grapevine culture took advantage of virgin soils that were more fertile in Etruria. In Greece, the geographic and climatic conditions (wind, drought, poor soil) determined
whether vines were on low trees or dry poles. In Etruscan territory, lush
vine shoots in the climate better suited to agriculture grew lavishly and

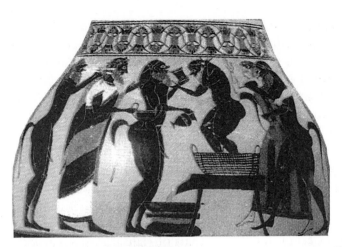

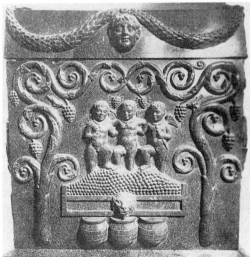

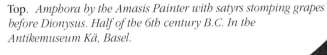

Top. *Amphora by the Amasis Painter with satyrs stomping grapes before Dionysus. Half of the 6th century B.C. In the Antikemuseum Kä, Basel.*

Left. *Cupids crushing grapes. St. Costanza sarcophagus. In the Vatican Museums, Vatican City.*

Red-figured Apulian vase shaped like a horn. Second half of the 4th century B.C. In a private collection.

blended harmoniously with elm, poplar and maple, or leaned on arbors, seen in certain Etruscan tomb paintings of the 6th and 5th century B.C.

Wine imports from Phoenicia and the Greek island of Chios have been reported since the 7th century and all of the 6th century B.C. Wine amphoras found in patrician tombs from that period all come from abroad and have either Greek, Phoenician, or African trademarks. Sometime later, wine became an agricultural surplus and was exported to Sicily and to the Mediterranean transalpine Gaul. Locally made amphoras for internal transport and for wine export developed greatly, testifying to the more sensible and intensive farming. Wine even served as a trading good.

Etruscan wines were known in Greece at the time of Alexander the Great (3rd century B.C.); Dionysius of Halicarnassus considered it equal to Falernum or to wines from the Roman hills. Martial compared it to Tarragona wine from his native Spain, admitting, however, together with Horace and Perseus, that the Veio territory produced nothing but a weak rosé from thick lees and was only a little better than the fetid Vatican wine. For other classical authors, the best wine was made in the Luni territory, bordering on Liguria. The Statonia and Graviscae vineyards also seem to have been touched by Dionysus' hand because they produced excellent wine. This extremely diversified wine production could in part be the reason why the Greeks believed that the Etruscans were hardy drinkers. And wasn't it a certain Arunte from Chiusi who took revenge against his own country by inviting the Gauls to invade it and capture the land with so many vineyards? In fact, Titus Livius tells us that the Gauls:

Attracted by the sweetness and new pleasure of wine, crossed the alps and occupied the fields previously farmed by the Etruscans.

The Etruscans were fond of sweet muscat, the kind that went to ones head and got the guests drunk. The name *Apianae muscat* was probably not so much due to its sweet taste, a true gluttony for bees (apes), as to some wine maker named Appius; indeed a certain *Aviles Apianas* (Aulus Appianus) was known in Florence. The remarkable variety of grapes and their products bear witness to deep rooted wine-making on Etruscan soil, an ancient trade that used grafts to create crosses and hybrids, layered vines with different tendrils. The ever-present Pliny the Elder informs us that the *Murgentina* tendril was introduced to Campania from Sicily, where it took on the name Pompeiana. But the true apotheosis of this vine species occurs in the land of Chiusi, in the heart of Etruria, with fertile and gentle slopes that invite the grapevine to a lasting and fruitful alliance. Other local strains in the meantime announced their future wines, Chianti or Orvieto and others.

Pliny informs us about Etruscan wines:

> *In Etruria the grapes from Todi are particular and have been given various names: sopina in Florence, talpona, esiaca and conseminia in Arezzo. Talpona is dark and produce white wine. For esiaca the greater the harvest the better the wine. Conseminia is dark and produces a short lasting wine, but its grapes, which last longer, are good to eat.*

Even Dionysius of Halicarnassus has something to say:

> *The grapevines from the Albani hills, Etruscan and Falernian regions are among those to be admired because the land is rich in vineyards and can offer plentiful and excellent products with little work.*

Long live the grapevine.

Wine traders

The wine trade along the ancient Mediterranean routes was enormous. It reached its high point straddling the 2nd century B.C. and the 1st century A.D., when large cargo ships cut through the Mediterranean heading for markets in the Roman empire. The great number of shipwrecks along these wine routes confirms this; as do the wine amphoras in the entire western Mediterranean region, not only on the coastline, but also along the riverbanks that lead inland, sometimes even beyond the English Channel. Roman wine had even reached England.

Such a heavy demand for wine from markets in Gaul must have made central and southern Italian wine-makers proud, because it paid tribute to the quality of their products. But there is reason to believe that at that time there was a sort of trade agreement to defend the great quantity of wine produced in those regions for export. The Roman senate planned well (many senators were landowners) to pass a law towards the end of the 2nd century (129 B.C.) that prohibited the inhabitants of Gaul from planting new grapes, with the exception for Roman citizens residing there. The measure failed to have the desired effect and the vineyards flourished in those regions.

Roman economic imperialism needed many trade routes to export and import products all the way to Rome. What better way was there, than by sea. Most of the provinces, or at least those that counted, were bathed by this sea. And it was already known that all goods could be packed in the holds, great loads such as marble obelisks, columns, tubs, sarcophagi, as well as less bulky materials like cloth, foodstuffs, glass, precious stones or ceramics. The practical Romans got their sums right: it cost much more to move a load of grain by land for a few hundred kilometers (wagons could only go about three kilometers in an hour) than send it from one end of the empire to the other by ship. If the ship was therefore unlucky enough to get caught in a gale, the loss would be compensated by the arrival of thousands of other ships that traveled the trade routes every year.

Only the foodstuffs contained in the amphoras and in sealed containers have survived wreckage. Contrary to what people think, grain traveled in coarse sacks or was shoveled into the hold and piled to balance the rest of the cargo. There is no trace of other foodstuffs, besides the bones of many pigs and the remains of ham bones found in a wreck from the 2nd century B.C. on the coast of Provence.

But amphoras were the true center of attention for these trading voyages. Thanks to them it has often been possible to find and recover shipwrecks that transported wine and other supplies. On several occasions, amphoras have gotten tangled in fishing nets. When reported, relatively easy recovery efforts have been started. According to reliable estimates, the number of amphoras carried must have been extremely high. On the Albenga wreck, for example, 11,000 wine amphoras were

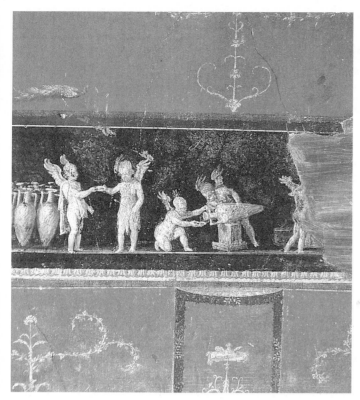

Cupids   pouring wine. Frieze from the great oecus in the Casa dei Vettii. Pompeii.

squeezed into the hold of this more than 40 meter long ship. The amphoras were piled in five vertical overlapping layers with the pointy bottoms of each amphora stuck into the space between four necks of the underlying amphoras. The space between the walls of the amphoras was packed with light and suitable pumice to absorb bumps and tossing during the long voyage.

Roman ships sailed to Gaul bringing nectar of the gods. The Roman wine amphoras were stamped on the rim with trade marks before being fired. In the wreck identified near Marseille, many of the 100 amphoras recovered had the name Sestius stamped on them, followed by various symbols among which an upside-down trident, an anchor, an ax, a star, a hook. Amphoras bearing the same marks as well as the name of a rich family in the region have been recovered at the site of ancient Cosa, today Ansedonia, on the Tyrrhenian coast about 100 km north of Rome.

The stories behind other shipwrecks are similar: amphoras and still more amphoras. No important wrecks have yet been found that have not given up their usual load of amphoras, of various tonnage and shape. For important cargo ships, up to 40 meters long and 12 to 15 meters wide, a load of 300-400 tons have been estimated. This estimate includes a large ship that capsized in Provence in the middle of the 1st century B.C. In that case, the many marked amphoras allowed experts to identify the exact place where both amphoras and wine were made. The name *Publius Veveius Papus*, together with others, is stamped on amphoras found near a kilm in Terracina, in lower Latium, a territory known for the production of Cecubum, one of the most renowned Roman wines. Together with Falernum, it made up the bulk of export.

Between Gaul and Rome intense trade existed even long after the conquest. The Gauls accepted the Roman lifestyle and, like the Romans, they ate while reclining on couches. Smoked ham and onions were loaded on ships that arrived in Rome and on the return voyage were laden with other trade goods: fruit trees from the Near East, peaches and apricots, but above all vineyard produce. The fertile districts of southern Gaul were right to grow grapevines. In a short time they produced great quality grapes, better even than Roman grapes. According to Cicero, wine was so appreciated by the Gauls that they drank it straight without cutting it with water. Soon this state of affairs led to a trade war that went badly for the Roman wine-makers, who appealed to the Emperor Domitian for protection. The diligent Emperor, ever ready to satisfy requests that favored Rome, grabbed the occasion of a wheat famine occurring at that same time, and with a decree in 91 A.D. ordered the vineyards to be cut down and substituted with wheat. Obviously the order regarded the Empire outside of Rome, and the province of Gaul in particular. Wanting to or not the Gauls obeyed. Beer and apple juice then took the place of wine to go with venison and boar, chicken and tuna that the Gauls continued to eat, but something important was missing. It wasn't until two centuries later that the legions of Probus came to restore the vineyards and extend the farming of *vitis vinifera* to other regions of northern Gaul.

The wine war has very ancient roots.

The Roman villas in the shadow of Mt. Vesuvius

Villas, upon which the peculiar Roman livelihood was based, were at the center of attention, especially along the Tyrrhenian coast between the 2nd century B.C. and 2nd century A.D.

The first rustic villas were built for farming. These were simple and uncluttered, answering exclusively to the needs of frugality and utility. According to a description by Seneca, the villa that belonged to Scipio Africanus at Liternum, in the beginning of the 2nd century B.C. was narrow, dimly lighted and bare. Scipio himself took care of the *fundus* (estate) where olives and grapes were grown. This corresponded with the simple life of the early farmers who Varro much later described as "typical of ancient times". A conspicuous blossoming of country villas has been recorded since the first half of the 2nd century B.C., especially in areas already strongly under Roman influence on the southern and western slopes of Massicum, in the Falernian plain, in the *Sinuessa* (today Mondragone) territory and in *Cales* (today Calvi Risorta).

Between the 2nd century B.C. and half of the 1st century B.C., they began to build country villas even in other areas, such as under Mt. Vesuvius, on the Sorrento peninsula, Sannio, Salerno, but most of all in the Phlaegrean fields calderon. The gentle and wholesome climate, the presence of fine warm springs, the Hellenist breeze that carried the steadfast traditions of Naples, all made the Campania shoreline one of the most sought after vacation lands for Roman nobility. The more illustrious figures in Roman aristocracy had villas on the seaside during the late republic: Marius, Silla, Pompeus, Caesar, Brutus, Cicero, Hortensius, Lucullus, Catullus, Varro who, among the elegant crowd at Baia and bustling Pozzuoli seaport, found all the characteristics of Rome (*illa pusilla Roma*).

The succession of villas and fishing villages was so dense that the geographer Strabo in the Augustan period wrote that the coast between Miseno Cape and Athenaeum Cape (the two extremities of Naples gulf) looked like one big city.

The seaside estates often included the farming of adjacent lands where livestock was bred, fisheries were created, and specialized nurseries were developed. Possession of a villa immediately became a new status symbol and because of their extravagance, procured for the landlord the nickname of *tritones* and *piscinarii*.

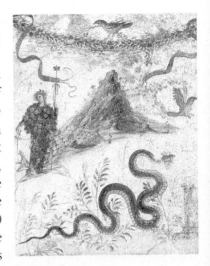

Nature in the Phlaegrean fields calderon ajusted to the invention of tools for the growing luxury of the Roman nobility. The rich businessman C. Sergius Orata became famous not only by inventing *balnea pensilia*, i.e., *suspensurae* baths, perhaps fed by the numerous smoking volcanoes in the area, but also for the *vivaria* (fisheries) dedicated to oysters and fish. These were particularly well suited for bays such as Lucrino or Fusaro or for pools built into the coast.

The residential villas on the slopes of Mt. Vesuvius and along the coast from Naples to Stabiae were often endowed with large tracts of productive land. Although incomplete, archeological investigations have often confirmed the presence of residential villas destined for farm labor, like the villa A of Oplontis. The oldest group of buildings rose next to a wine *torcularium*, substituted later by service buildings south of the large pool. Villa B was also endowed with residential quarters on the upper floors, while the inside portico housed the storerooms of a *negotiator vinarius*.

The coastal villas were matched in the fertile Vesuvian inland, on the plains and in the hills, by a tight network of country villas destined mostly to wine-making. This is confirmed by

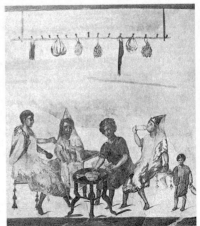

Top. *Bacchus and Mt. Vesuvius, drawn with a single cone (prior to the 79 A.D. eruption). Casa del Centenario, Pompeii.*

Fresco with a tavern scene. In the National Archeology Museum, Naples.

the widespread use of grapevines in
the entire area gravitating around Mt.
Vesuvius, including the higher slopes of
the mountain. The literary description by
Strabo and Martial have been confirmed
by archeological evidence. Starting from
the celebrated picture of *lararium* (a
place set aside for household deities)
in the House of the Centenary in
Pompeii with Mt. Vesuvius covered
with grapevines almost to the summit,
and Bacchus (Dionysus) at the foot
turned into a grape. He takes on the
typical gesture of holding up a thyrsus

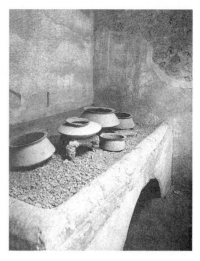

with one hand, while pouring a drink for a leopard with the other. The
early settlements around Mt. Vesuvius date to the 2nd century B.C. and,
like the rest of the Campania region, were primarily farms with no

Top. *Pots over the fire from the kitchen in the Casa dei Vettii, Pompeii.*

Facsimile of a wine press in the torcularium at Villa dei Misteri. Pompeii.

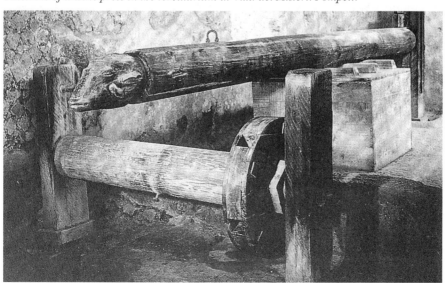

architectural pretensions, small bare rooms around a courtyard, and designed exclusively to take advantage of the farmland pertaining to the villa itself.

The residential quarters were designed for the landlord. His presence on the *fundus* contributed in a remarkable way to assuring that it was fruitful by his constant overseeing of the *familia rustica*. The main house was always separated from the rustic and servant huts (*pars rustica*). It had a domestic wing with a kitchen, storerooms, servant's quarters, stalls and livestock shelters, as well as the *pars fructuaria* sector set aside to prepare and preserve fresh produce, particularly grapes and to some extent olives. Each were handled with specialized equipment such as a wine screw press, a wine vat, and a oil press.

Wine making essentially required a *torcularium*, a place to crush grapes and press the seeds and skins, and a wine cell to ferment the grape must. The first was a tub for crushing (*forum* or *calcatorium*) *pedibus calcantibus* (with bare feet) lined with crockery and equipped with a window to quickly unload a chest full of grapes, and a handling room. There the ancient screw press was set up (or two for a big farm such as Villa Pisanella) one such operation, as described by Cato, was reconstructed in the *torcularium* at the Villa of Mysteries in Pompeii. The wine screw press was invented by the Greeks (*torcula graecanica*) and has been in use through modern times.

The rugged wine screw was made from a sturdy trunk (*prelum*) that became the fulcrum on a support beam (*arbor*) attached to the floor and was lowered unto the mass of seeds and skins by a winch (*sucula*) implanted between two beams (*stipites*), these also attached to the ground. It all worked by lever (*vectes*). To assure that the machine was stable, two small holes were dug in the ground in front of two square stones pierced by the lever, to work the *stipites* and beside the forced lever stone to work the *arbor*.

The *torcularium* of the so-called Villa 6 in Terzigno offers an interesting example of the way grape must was collected and decanted. It flowed through a drainage channel in the bottom of the pressing tub, along two walls that formed banks to keep the juice from spilling, and ended in a huge lead pipe (*fistula*). The juice flowed into the adjacent collecting cistern (*lacus*) so perfectly sealed and endowed with a de-

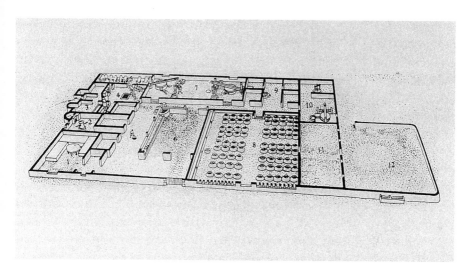

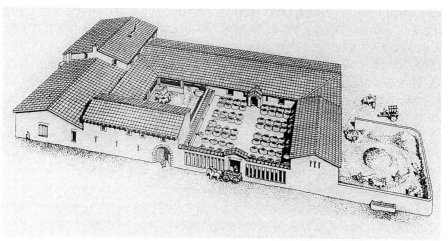

Hypothetical model of the Pisanella Villa at Boscoreale. 1 triclinium, 2 oven, 3 baths, 4 kitchen, 5 stall, 6 courtyard, 7 room for crushing grapes, 8 courtyard for fermenting the grape must, 9 rooms for servants, 10 room for pressing olives, 11 granary, 12 threshing-floor.

canting vat at the bottom. From here the must was poured into a tub dug into the marble crest of the opposite wall. This was also completely lined with plaster *signinum*. From here the juice flowed through two lead pipes into fermentation tubs.

Following the tradition of the Campania region, the wine cell was left uncovered or protected by roofing. It was contained in terracotta containers (*dolia*) sunk into the dirt to their necks (*dolia defossa*) in parallel rows. Paths were usually left to cross the room. These containers were sealed by a flat clay lid called *operculum*. A second cover placed over it was shaped like a terracotta disk (*tectorium*).

Roman agronomists furnish a good deal of information on plant set-up and equipment that one would expect to find on a farm that grows grapes and olives. According to Cato, for a one hundred *iugeri* surface area (25 hectares) a vineyard needed ten laborers to plow (*bovarii*), to transport (*asinarii*), to slop the pigs. What's more, a farm needed two oxen and two donkeys for the wagon (*plaustrum*), a donkey for the grist mill (*mola*), two wine screws, two *dolia* able to hold the yield of five harvests, twenty *dolia* for the dregs of grapes, twenty for wheat, lids for the *dolia*, three plows, harnesses for the beasts of burden and draught along with a certain number of iron farming tools such assickles, shovels and hoes. The use of such tools illustrates the typical concept that farms had to be as much as possible self-sufficient.

The Vesuvian country villas are the best preserved in the Campania region, thanks to their burial at the 79 A.D. eruption. They have given us back tools described in literary sources, mostly for wine making, but to some extent also oil, as well as other produce like wheat, fruit, legumes and vegetables for the home table, all found carbonized. These products were the *circa villam* crops, grown near the villa within fences (*horti*). There were also fields of grass (clover, purple medic, wild peas) for stock animals. Large open-air areas closed in by low walls where hay was dried, were common on these farms.

From the vineyard to the table

Since antiquity, the area around Mt. Vesuvius has been covered with lush vineyards that climbed even the highest slopes of the volcano. The importance of wine-making in the life of Pompeii's inhabitants can readily be seen by looking at the cupids engaged in vintage portrayed in the well known frescos at the Casa dei Vettii.

The array of Campania wines during Roman times is broad with a number of vintages (*Aminea, Calventina, Falerna, Gemina minor Holconia, Murgentina-Pompeiana, Vennuncula*). In the area around Pompeii, at least four of these prospered. According to Pliny, Murgentina was the number one grape grown. This originally came from Sicily, but took so well to Pompeii that it developed the name *Pompeiana*. Again Pliny and Columella remind us that *Gemina minor*, thrived on Mt. Vesuvius and on the Sorrento mountains. This is a grapevine from the *Aminea* strain that was held to be noble, but provided low yields. It is very likely that the slopes of Mt. Vesuvius were planted with *Aminea* grapes, whereas *Murgentina* thrived on the plain near Pompeii. *Holconia* was also grown. These grapes were named after a family from Pompeii that was growing in popularity. Another grape, called *Vennuncula*, filled the Sarno plain and grew all the way to Sorrento. Both grapes were poor quality (third choice). Columella, Celsus and Pliny all mentioned them for the quantity of juice produced and not for their quality.

All around Pompeii there were various kinds and qualities of wine, from those for everyday use, made from the vineyards growing on the plains, to the finest wines from the slopes of Mt. Vesuvius. The *Vesuvinum* or *Vesvinum* have been found on three of Pompeii's amphoras and one from Carthage. Perhaps they are the forerunners of *Lacryma Christi*, and the famous *Pompeianum* that, according to Pliny, did not improve in the first ten years of aging and caused headache.

The most widely used farming technique employed by Vesuvian vineyards was bracing the grape wines up on supports, such as growing them on rectangular arbors almost forming a roof (*vitis compluviata*). This technique, one of the six listed by Pliny the Elder, was particularly advantageous and convenient in hot and dry places, such as around Mt. Vesuvius, because the leaves formed a kind of canopy that shaded the soil and kept it cool. Still used today, this vineyard technique is recorded in land adjacent to the country villa of Boscoreale, in the so-called *Forum Boarium* (cattle market). Here the grapevines were planted four Roman feet apart (each foot = 29.59 cm). Columella suggested that the framework of the grape arbor was about five feet off the ground and never more than seven and no less than four feet. Varro argued that ideally a vineyard should be as high as a man is tall.

Pliny felt that the height of a crossbeam should depend on the altitude of the vineyard. Very likely, just as today, the arbor poles were chestnut, an expensive but plentiful wood in the area. Chestnut poles lasted at least ten years and were preferable, according to Columella, to poplar which lasted no more than two years.

The vineyard received care year-round. The grapevines were planted in straight rows with shoots rising up on poles. The ground around the base of the vine was tilled several times a year with a two-pronged spade. Plants were pruned, roots jutting to the surface were cut, poles were set back in place or substituted when necessary.

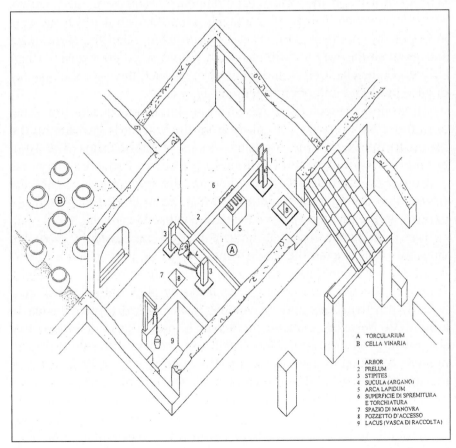

A TORCULARIUM
B CELLA VINARIA

1 ARBOR
2 PRELUM
3 STIPITES
4 SUCULA (ARGANO)
5 ARCA LAPIDUM
6 SUPERFICIE DI SPREMITURA
   E TORCHIATURA
7 SPAZIO DI MANOVRA
8 POZZETTO D'ACCESSO
9 LACUS (VASCA DI RACCOLTA)

Layout of a torcularium in a country villa at Terzigno. A torcularium, B wine cellar.

Once the grapes ripened, towards the end of September, the harvest began. Pliny and Varro mentioned that the grape harvest lasted from September 24th to November 11th, whereas Columella coincided the start of the wine harvest with the appearance of the constellation of Virgo on September 28th. In their farm calendar the Latin agronomists recommended that preparation begin in the storeroom forty days before the grape harvest. The large, deep terracotta containers (*dolia defossa*) had to be scraped, washed and covered on the inside with pitch, preferably from Bruzium, to assure that they wouldn't leak. In the attempt to improve the bouquet, sometimes compromised by the pitch, resin was added.

Next they made sure the wine screw press was assembled correctly and in working order. Parts of the press, the large oak lever (*prelum*), the upright posts *stipites*, the winch (*sucula*), and the shaft (*arbor*), were taken down from the attic where they were hung after the last harvest to safeguard them from the damp floor. The pulleys were greased and the ropes rewound. Finally, the crushing tub was carefully cleansed. They never overlooked the inspection of the harvesting tools, the small curved knives (*falculae vineaticae, ungues ferrei*), the wicker baskets (*corbulae*), and the loading wagons (*plaustra*).

Atoning sacrifices were made to Dyonisus/Bacchus, protector of the press and the wine, whose image was jealously guarded in the *lararium* within the *torcularium*. Finally, they began the harvest, carried out by servants and day laborers hired locally; children were given the chore of picking up the fallen grapes. Filled to the brim with grapes, the baskets were carried on a cart to the villa and unloaded by hand into the crushing tub through a window. The grapes were crushed with bare feet: the juice ran into the collecting tub (*lacus*) or into the *dolia* where it began to decant. The dregs were placed in a basket (*fiscellae*) and pressed in turn by being placed under the oak lever that was lowered by the *torcularii* increasing the pressure on the mass of pits and skins, winding the ropes that passed over the head of the oak lever by the strength of pulley leverage (*vectes*).

After the pressing, the dregs ended up in the *dolia* to be used for food preservatives or to fashion a drink (*lora*) mostly given to slaves in the wintertime. Next they boiled down a small portion of the must in a bronze caldron (*cortinale*) to get a sugary concentrate (*defritum* or *defrutum*) used to preserve food, give wine a higher proof, or for other products such as *sapa* and *caroenum* used as a syrup to preserve fruit. The remaining must was poured into the *dolia* of the wine cellar.

The fermentation process lasted for nine days. The *dolia* were capped with their own lids (*opercula*). They were sealed around the mouth with clay, mud or Bruzium resin to make sure air would not deteriorate the wine. As an additional protection against the heat and rain, because the wine cellar was often exposed, *opercula* were covered by terracotta shingles (*tectoria*) resting on three legs. Pliny the Elder recommended opening the *dolia* in winter on mild days, when the south wind was calm (Austrum) and there was no full moon.

The best wines were left to age in the *dolia*. This process could be accelerated after decanting, by placing the amphoras in predetermined places on the upper floors or even above the kitchen where the warmth and smoke were usually taken advantage of to season wood. Columella advised using a normal attic because he believed that the excessive heat could ruin the wine. This procedure was not applied to everyday Pompeian wines that had to be drunk within the year. Vesuvinum and Pompeianum were the only ones that improved with aging, but no more than ten years. It is now certain that *vinum odoratum* was also made in Pompeii's suburb. This wine was treated with fragrant herbs (*odoramenta*) that did not appeal to all tastes.

The wine made in the countryside around Pompeii was for local consumption and export. Judging from the few transport amphoras found in most of the country villas investigated, wine selling was not done by the producers, but by designated merchants (*negotiatores* or *mercatores vinarii*) who traveled about the villas filling goatskins (*utres*) or with the *culleus*, a wagon holding an immense oxen skin sack, equivalent to twenty amphoras (about 524 liters). The *negotiators* could buy the grapes while still on the vine, and oversee the harvest. Finally, they saw to the distribution in local or distant markets.

One example of a building used by a *negotiator vinarius* is Villa B of Oplontis, where more than 400 wine transport amphoras have been found in the arms of the peristyle.

8 The olive tree

The legend of the olive tree

The origin of the olive tree and its oil has been passed down to us by myths and legends. The olive tree has been sacred and essential for millennia. It is a symbol that appears in every major event of life. It has been chiseled and painted in ancient rock drawings or paintings. It has come to symbolize abundance, peace and renewed life. What other tree besides the olive can symbolize the culture, the human activity and the luxuriant nature found in the Mediterranean basin?

The Greeks said that olive trees were a gift from Athena. Homer narrates that Odysseus fashioned his wedding bed from a gigantic olive trunk. One Greek legend has it that to put an end to squabbling between Athena and Poseidon for control of Attica, Zeus promised the land in prize to whoever could offer the most useful gift. Poseidon struck the ground with his trident, creating a splendid horse. Athena instead made an olive tree. Olive oil was shown to be such an important food, medicine and source of light that Zeus bestowed the victory and Attica upon Athena.

Greek mythology attributes the discovery of the olive tree to the god of agriculture, Aristaeus. He was the son of Apollo and Cyrene. Akropus, who was the mythical founder of Athens, was venerated for having taught the Greeks how to extract olive oil after receiving knowledge of the tree from Aristaeus.

The olive tree was sacred and revered in Athens. The Athenians venerated the sacred olives from the tree that the goddess herself germinated on the Acropolis. Anyone who damaged the tree received the death penalty in early times. At a later date the punishment was exile and confiscation of property. The olive cult was so important that even the land they grew on was considered sacred. What's more, only virgins and chaste men were permitted to grow them.

The Romans attributed the olive to the goddess Minerva. As goddess of wisdom, she had taught men how to grow it. The wild olive was, however, attributed to Heracles, who it is said struck the ground hard with a stick and made roots grow. Another legend says that Romulus and Remus, the founders of Rome, were born beneath an olive tree, then put into a chest and thrown into the Tiber River. The chest was tossed ashore near the Palatine Hill. There a wolf suckled the twins.

Olive oil in ancient times

Olive oil has been an important foodstuff for the Mediterranean population since remote times.

Olive farming dates back more than 6000 years. Much evidence points to Syria as the birthplace, where the Semitic tribes farmed it. From there it traveled to Egypt, Asia Minor and finally Greece. It appears that the Phoenicians introduced it to South Italy, the lands of the future Roman Empire and then the entire Mediterranean. The spread of olives and olive oil production from the eastern to western Mediterranean lands was the work of traders. Olives were first carried aboard ships from Mycenae, then Phoenicia, Etruria and Greece to South Italy, the coasts of Liguria, France and Spain.

As in ancient times, the olive tree grows up to 40 miles inland on the coast of the Mediterranean. For thousands of years, olives have been a major cash crop for Mediterranean cultures. The large containers crammed into buildings dating to the Minoan and Mycenaean period bear witness of such cultivation, as do the many oil amphoras found along major shipping lanes in the Mediterranean Sea.

In ancient times, olive oil was common to all Mediterranean cuisines. People with distant lifestyles shared the same food ingredients grown on the soil dampened by the *mare nostrum*.

Olive oil as a condiment has been passed down from civilization to civilization, and the ability to transform a thorny shrub with bitter berries into a tree yielding precious oil has been the work of many people over the centuries.

Ab antiquo, the olive tree was grown and praised for its oil in Syria, in Palestine and in Crete. Because the Phoenicians were considered the best navigators and shrewdest merchants from the 2nd millennium B.C. onwards, they are credited for having exported the olive tree from Lebanon to the coastal regions of the Mediterranean Sea, and for bringing this "liquid gold" to everyone's attention.

The understanding that olive oil and other seed oils are indispensable lipids has been known since the 3rd millennium B.C. in Syria and Palestine. The remains of implements used to make oil, along with pieces of large containers to hold it, have been found in the Bronze Age strata at Ugarit.

Silver skyphos from the Casa del Menandro at Pompeii. In the National Archeology Museum, Naples.

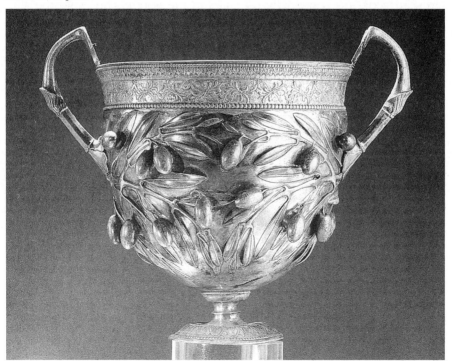

The Bible mentions that 20 *Kor* (each *Kor* is equal to 450 liters) of olive oil squeezed per year was among the foodstuffs sent to Hiram, king of Tyros, by Salomon in exchange for construction materials and craftsmen to build the temple. Again the Bible reports that Joshua and Zorababel furnished oil to the Phoenicians of Sidon and Tyros in exchange for precious Lebanon cedar. The olives remaining on the branches were left for the indigent, while the best oil was destined for food sacrifices, as an ingredient in *focaccia* bread, and filled the properly arranged jars in regal pantries.

At the end of Phoenician colonization, the signs of that civilization remained long impressed on Sicily. It is believed that the skill in growing olive trees came to Rome from Sicily, after first passing through the Campania region. Pliny the Elder states that the art of oil production reached Rome by way of the Etruscans, who traded heavily with the Phoenicians. Grapevines and olive trees had a huge impact on the Etruscan economy, especially on cities in the South. They sold the surplus and reaped great profit. On the shipwreck found near the Giglio island and dating to 600 B.C., olives preserved in brine have been found in the Etruscan transport amphoras. Olive pits have been found in the Tomb of the Olives at Cerveteri (575-550 B.C.). They are to be considered food offerings to the deceased. In one passage, Cato refers to olives as food for slaves. It is thus even correct to think of olives as a source of good quality protein.

According to other sources, the olive tree came to Etruria by way of Greece. The Etruscan word *eleiva* meant oil and derived from the Doric-Greek *elaiva*. The Latin word *amurca* (oil dregs) came from the Greek *amorga*. This cannot be explained without considering that the *o* changes to the *u* sound and the *g* becomes *c* in Etruscan.

Because it was good to eat high on the hog, wine and oil were brought to Italy and to Etruria between the end of the 8th and beginning of the 7th century B.C. The amphoras carrying both wine and oil were made in Attica, where olive tree plantations were well established. Olive farming arrived sometime later in Etruria. Besides its value as a foodstuff, oil was already used as a base to prepare balms and ointments. It was rarely used as a fuel for lanterns.

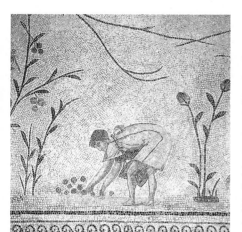

Mosaic with olive gathering. 3rd-4th century A.D. In the Bardo Museum, Tunis.

Unloading amphoras from one ship to another. Floor mosaic from Piazzale delle Corporazioni. 1st century A.D. Old Ostia.

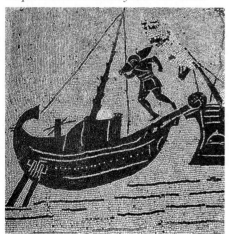

Despite the fact that olives are still grown throughout Greece, the tree has never been intensively farmed. The trees are often grown along the edges of fields or roads, or scattered through the countryside. The ancient Greeks obtained different qualities of oil from green olives (*omphakion*), the first press of dark olives, and finally ordinary oil. The oldest rotating oil mill, the antecedent of the *trapetum* found at Pompeii, was discovered in the city of Olynthus.

The Greek colonies of Messina and Crotone had olive leaves and branches stamped onto their coins. This is proof that the olive tree was widespread in southern Italy by the 5th century B.C. The commercial contacts between the Greek colonies and Romans favored olive tree farming around Rome.

The Romans praised the olive tree. Columella defined it as a "prime tree". It was grown so extensively during the Roman Empire that entire provinces of Spain and North Africa were converted into olive tree plantations. Pliny the Elder lists the various types of olives known at that time and already believed to have existed at an earlier age. Among these were the very rare and sweeter than raisin olives grown in Africa and in Spain.

In the beginning, the Romans flavored their foods with pork fat (lard), but the connoisseurs who found that taste a little harsh, with time turned their attention to more refined substances, such as the famous pheasant fat that Apicius recommended for frying. Lard was called *adeps suillus* or more simply *adeps* by the Romans. They used it fresh or after saving it for some time. The Romans believed that adding fat to vegetable soup derived from the Greeks.

In Cato one can see how this has survived in the ancient ingredient of lard in cakes, especially the so-called *globi* (a kind of sponge cake) made from semolina and cheese and then fried in fat, called *unguentum*. This was also an ingredient in *encytum* and *mustacei*, the pastries based on wine must.

With the spread of olive tree farming, olive oil became the principle fat in Roman cooking. Animal fat fell into disuse except on pauper's tables and by farmers living in the provinces far from the olive oil producing centers.

Cato, Pliny, Columella and the most famous Latin agricultural writers of the time left their teachings on olive tree farming and oil making. They gave precise instructions on how to make it and the different kinds of oil that could be obtained, as well as preserving methods. The oil flowing from the press was thick. To thin it and keep it from coagulating they heated the room. Because they used wood fires, the oil and honey often smelled like smoke. Sometimes, depending on the season, it was enough to face the room south into the sun to capture the heat. Experts agreed that this was best means of guaranteeing fine oil. Within the ruins of Villa Pisanella, on the slopes of Mt. Vesuvius, there is an interesting example of an oil press in a room heated by sunlight.

There were several kinds of oil in that period of history. There was summer oil (*oleum acerbum*) made from fallen green olives. The best oil (*oleum omphacium*) was made in September. Green oil (*oleum viride*) was pressed in December from fallen black olives. Virgin olive oil (*oli flos*) came from the first light squeeze, while *oleum sequens* flowed from the second heavier squeeze. Ordinary oil (*oleum cibarium*) came from still another pressing and cost four-fold less than virgin olive oil. *Cibarium* was used more in the kitchen, whereas virgin oil was saved for salad dressing because of its high cost.

Unfortunately, because oil was not highly refined and received no special treatment to prolong freshness, it went rancid very fast. For this reason it was salted, or the olives themselves were saved as long as possible to be squeezed at a moment's notice for fresh oil year-round. In this case, they picked the olives from the trees while still green and placed them under oil. The best oils were produced in the land of

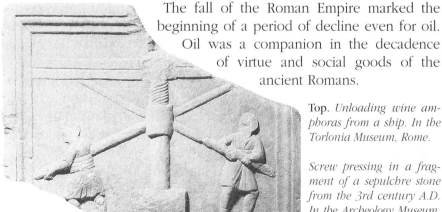

Venafro and Liburnia.

Besides being used for food, oil was used for illumination, as an ointment for athletes, as a cosmetic and as a cure-all. Oil from wild trees became medicine. They also used oils from other fruits, such as mirth for wine, and walnut and almond oil. These, however, were never used in the kitchen.

When Rome was in its glory, at the beginning of the decadent period, the Augustan colonies in Molise, settled after the extermination of the Samnites by Silla (87 B.C.), prospered so that they acquired the rank of municipalities. Their coins were at that time stamped with the effigy of Minerva holding an olive branch in her hand.

The fall of the Roman Empire marked the beginning of a period of decline even for oil. Oil was a companion in the decadence of virtue and social goods of the ancient Romans.

Top. *Unloading wine amphoras from a ship. In the Torlonia Museum, Rome.*

Screw pressing in a fragment of a sepulchre stone from the 3rd century A.D. In the Archeology Museum, Aquileia.

The art of making oil

The art of making oil is ancient. The creativity and skills of ancient peoples were brought to bear on designing machinery and in time perfecting it. Numerous finds in Asia Minor and along the banks of the Mediterranean Sea allow us to trace the evolution of oil making through the different societies that have resided there.

The first oil was made by squeezing olives by hand, or stamping on them with bare feet. After all, it worked with wine. For example, in some north African areas, special wooden sandals were used. On Crete and in Egypt the art of oil making already underwent enormous change thanks to the invention of the mortar. At first, this was made out of concave stones in which the olives were pounded by hand. The mash was then transferred to a stone tub, where hot water caused to oil to rise to the surface. Once separated, the oil could be skimmed off and placed into jars.

The mortar was the first tool used to make oil. It was shaped like a bowl and pounded with a round stone pestle. The mash was placed on a flat stone and surrounded by a crown of breaded olive branches. This kept the mash from running over the sides during the pressing. Two or three large stones, one on top of the other, were used to press the olive mash. The oil that flowed from this was collected in clay pots below.

Oil technology dates back to the 2nd millennium with the invention of the stone mill for mashing and the lever to multiply the pressing force. The Romans perfected two types of olive mills: the *trapetum*, with two round stones that crushed the olives against the walls of the tub, and the vertical rotating mill that crushed the olives against the floor of the tub.

The Romans made a leap forward in olive oil technology in the 1st century B.C. with the *trapetum* and the screw press. The former was expensive and used exclusively by large land holdings. The cone-shaped stone mortar served the less important olive growers with small parcels of land. The screw press made the big difference for mashing.

The Romans used a lever to crush the mash. This was a large pole attached to the wall that pressed layer upon layer of oil mash. Until the discovery of the vertical press in Liguria in the 17th century, this remained the time tested technology.

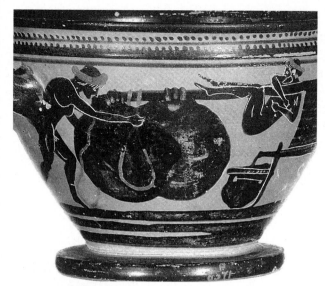

Black-figured skyphos with grape pressing. Half of the 6th century B.C. In the Museum of Fine Arts, Boston.

For the first three centuries of the Empire, the province of Betica provided amphoras for transporting oil. This is likely because the Baetis Valley (Guadalquivir) had immense olive groves that produced oil for most of the Roman Empire. Mills were located along water routes. The loaded oil amphoras were sent down river to seaports, then shipped to Rome where they were emptied and then destroyed. It cost less to destroy them because they were so hard to clean. The quarter of Testaccio (*mount of crocks*) in Rome was built on millions of pieces of Spanish amphoras. It is an example of the largest monumental archive in the history of Imperial Roman commerce.

At the time of the great technological boom, Roman olive growers were faced with an architectural problem. How should an olive oil refinery be built? Columella, who was considered an authority, said that the edifice ought to be built in a sunny place, away from the cold north wind. A mild temperature was indispensable because it favored oil extraction. Warm oil flows and cold oil condenses. Columella disapproved of cellar mills because he believed that poor ventilation would ruin the oil.

Making fine quality oil required great skill, a technology in constant evolution and sunny, well-ventilated environments. In the Mediterranean basin, the art of man was in harmony with the bountifulness of nature.

Several written records have come down to us regarding the quality of some oils. The oldest were written by Cato the Elder, who already at the beginning of the 2nd century B.C. in his celebrated *De Agri Cultura*, recognized Venafro as having the best olives. He indicated the best way to sell olives. Indeed, he refers to the way Venafro handled olives and how this spread to the entire Roman world.

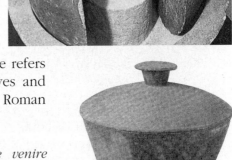

> *Oleam pendentem hac lege venire oportet: olea pendens in fundo venafro venibit. (The hanging olive needs to be sold following this rule: the hanging olive will be sold in the land of Venafro).*

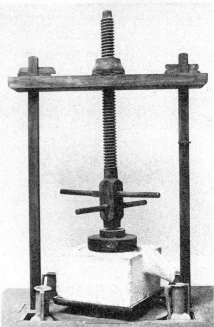

Top. *Facsimile of a wheat or olive grinding stone. In the Museum of Roman Civilization, Rome.*

Small vase (aryballos) in bucchero for perfumes. The inscription (aska mi eleivana) tells us that it contained oil (I am an oil phile). In the Real Collegio Carlo Alberto, Moncalieri.

Bottom. *Facsimile of an olive screw press (torcularium olearium). In the Museum of Roman Civilization, Rome.*

In *De Re Rustica,* Varro praises the quality of olive oil with the following words:

> *Quod far comparem Campano? Quod triticum Appulo? Quod vinum Phalerno? Quod oleum Venafrano? (What spelt could compare to that of Campania? What wheat to that from Apulia? What wine to Falernian? What oil to that from Venafro?).*

In his *Satirae,* Horace gives the highest praise to Venafro's oil (*pressa quod bacca remisit olivae*). The poet informed us that the first press olives from Venafro (*quod prima Venafri pressit cella*), were mixed with others, probably to improve it.

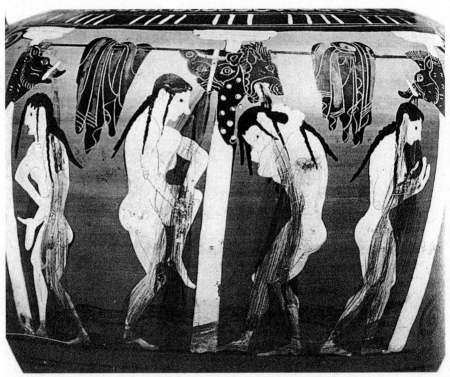

Detail from a Corinth vase with young women washing. The streams of water flow from lion and boar heads. 6th century B.C. In the Staatliche Museen, Berlin.

9 Exercise and body care

The palaestra

The Greek taste for exercise and physical activity had ancient roots. The funeral games celebrated in honor of Patroclus by the wailing Achilles in the Iliad, the palace games of Alcinoo and the attempt to pull Odysseus bow on Ithaca, described in the Odyssey, give us a sense of this interest. By the time Troy fell (about 1300 B.C.), the valorous Greek warriors, Achilles' companions, had become athletes. They inherited the belief that exercise was fundamental to become good combatants. This attitude was consolidated in the culture at that time and thereafter. At the LXV Olympic games (circa 520 B.C.), a new competition was inaugurated where worriers clad in battle dress raced.

Although legend has it that Hercules started the Olympic games to celebrate the memory of Pelops, the more accredited tradition honors Iphytus, king of Hellas. At that time in 776 B.C., a terrible epidemic was ravaging the population of the Peloponnesus. Were the gods in some way angry? The oracle made a suggestion to the king that was perhaps unusual, but would work. He recommended that games be held at the site where the epidemic struck and dedicated then to the gods. These deities would take pleasure in being honored by the most beautiful, healthy and strongest youths around, pumped up for the competition and yearning to win. Weren't the gods driven by the same emotions as mankind? How could they be anything but enthralled by such a demonstration of strength and virility? The epidemic soon abated, as a sign of the gods' benevolence for humankind and the games. Since then, whenever the Greeks built a city, the theater and the stadium have stood out.

With all likelihood, Greek children began physical training by age twelve, but what a difference between Sparta and Athens. Plutarch tells us that young Spartan boys learned reading and writing, but without achieving great proficiency. Their main education was:

To learn to obey, endure difficulties and win battles.

The twelfth birthday heralded trials and tribulations. Heads were shaved. They received only one mantel per year, a straw mattress, little water for washing and very little oil for balm. They were whipped for even slight infractions. They were given just a few crumbs to eat so as to stimulate daring and guile that only comes from pilfering food from others when you are hungry. It was a wretched life to belong to the state until death, often reached prematurely in those conditions.

Athenian youths had it somewhat easier, especially when fathers could provide an education, a pedagogue, side by side with a trainer who taught physical fitness. When the money was unavailable, farming could improve the body and soul. According to Xenophon:

Rising early and being forced to do manual labor in the fields conferred manly vigor on youths...The land incites farmers to bear arms in defense of their country, because his harvests are the spoils of the strongest, available to all...

Young Athenian women lived in recluse. They were hardly allowed to get a breath of fresh air in the courtyard. No men were to gaze upon them, not even the males of the household could touch them. Their entire education took place indoors. Physical education was not part of their curriculum. They learned to do housework, spin wool, sew, make clothes, and sweeten their temperament through music and literature. Experienced women and mothers guided them.

Spartan girls, on the other hand, played sports in public like boys. Their short garments scandalized Euripides:

Outdoors with young men, with their legs bare and clothes waving.

Spartan girls grew vigorously. They were wrestlers, expert javelin and discus throwers. Here too, the City-state came first. Healthy and strong young women would one day become mothers of large robust families. They would be able to bring up future soldiers in the best possible way. Even Lycurgus was a convinced defender of these principles:

> *Get young women used to parading nude in processions just like men, to dancing and singing at religious ceremonies, to the presence and gazes of the young men.*

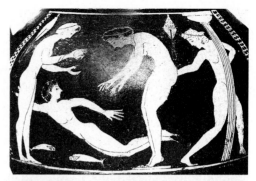

On red figured vases (end of the 5th century B.C.) we find depictions of gymnasts bearing exercise equipment. We even have the name of one gymnast, the mythical Atalanta who adored the goddess Artemis. She was a model for young athletic

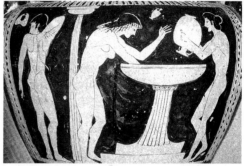

Top. *Amphora by the Andokides Painter: the swimmers. Last quarter of the 6th century B.C. In the Louvre, Paris.*

Crater painted in the Göttingen Painter style. A woman scrapes her back with a strigil, while two others wash. First decade of the 5th century B.C. In the Museo Civico, Bari.

women who trained the body while invoking the protection of the goddess. Another picture reveals typical gymnast equipment, such as the sponge, a round oil vase and the strigil to scrape off sweat after a workout. It is likely that even young Athenian women had public or private space set aside for body care. Portrayals of women splashing in monumental fountains, or swimming, washing and grooming suggest open areas outside the home. They lead us to think of gymnasiums or more delightful places where athletes could freely dedicate themselves to physical exercise. Since Hellenistic times, public baths and gymnasiums have been reserved to women on certain days.

The *palaestra* was consecrated to physical fitness. It was a square piece of land set aside with walls all around, but no roof. Rooms along one side served for changing. There were also rooms for bathing, for resting, holding sports equipment, oil and sand. The god Hermes (Mercury) was the ever vigil patron of gymnasts. His busts decorated the *palaestra*. The space established for sports had a boundary stone to mark the start or finish lines of a race, or trees arranged in the open air. Wells were also nearby, where water could be drawn from the ground to fill great tubs for bathing. Athletic equipment like sponges for washing, ampoules for oil and strigils to scrape away sweat could be found throughout the area.

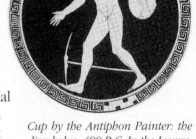

Gymnasts trained hard, not just to avoid an instructors anger, but to avoid the wrath of his long forked stick used on the lazy or clumsy. Capable young men who were enthusiastic and skilled might dream of becoming professional athletes. They would be admired and cheered by all. Winners of the most important tournaments, the Panhellenic or even the Olympic games, could expect to eat for free at the public mess hall of their city, and sit in the best seats at the theater, and more than anything else be remembered over the ages for their prowess on the field.

Cup by the Antiphon Painter: the discobolus. 490 B.C. In the Louvre, Paris.

Cup by the Thalia Painter with javelin thrower. 520 B.C. In the Louvre, Paris.

The trainers tried to follow the rules established by Aristotle, recommending that youths play all sports to get a good all-round training, instead of pushing them to set a record in only one discipline.

Athletes competed naked (*gimnos*) and rubbed themselves down with oil

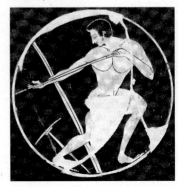

before competing. With the following words, Thucydides, tells us how this practice was inherited from Sparta:

> *The Lacedaemonians were the first to show themselves nude and appear in public without clothes. They used oil for sporting events. At one time, the athletes used a kind of belt to hide their genitals even at the Olympic games.*

Pausanias tells us that this occurred before Orsippos from Megara let his jock strap fall because it was easier to move without it in a race. He would have likely won the race anyway, but this coincidence was enough to change the custom.

A bath in the fountain, or in the tub at the *palaestra* if it had one, was required before exercising. Then came the rubdown with oil brought from home in a small flask (*alabastron*). After, sand was strewn which attached to the oil, forming a thin layer to protect the body from the elements. When exercises were over, the oil and sand that had hardened from sweat and dust were removed by the curved bronze strigil. Finally, athletes took another bath and went home or elsewhere.

The games

The word *palaestra* derives from the ancient and noble sport of wrestling (*palé*). Before the bout, children using hoes would begin to till the soil where they might fall. This tool is often depicted on vases representing sporting events. The tilling alone was a healthy exercise. Then the boys would face each other, two at a time with their heads lowered and their arms thrust out in front of them attempting to strike and grip their adversary's arm, neck or trunk. It was the trainer's job to teach them all the holds. During competitions, fighters were matched by drawing broad beans with letters written on them (two with a, two with b, two with c, and so on).

There were different kinds of races. The single sprint around a stadium (about 180 meters), twice around a stadium (*diaulos*), or four times around the stadium (*hippios*), and the long-distance race (24 stadiums, about 4 kilometers). The distance was a round trip between the starting line designated by the boundary stones (sawed off columns) and the end of the track. At the other end of the stadium, the runner rounded a boundary stone (*terma*) and returned to the starting line to begin again if the race was a long one. The runners waited on their feet, chest forward and feet close together for the starting signal.

For long jumping, young athletes would began by examining the place they would fall after the jump. To increase their distance they used *haltares*, which were hollow stone or lead tools weighing from 1 to 5 kilograms and shaped like half moons to fit into the palm of a hand. They had two weights with a handle bar to be gripped between them. With one weight held in each hand, and arms slightly bent, the athletes began their sprint. As they leaped they snapped their arms backward and then forward. With that technique they were able to jump a distance of 15 meters. The unsurpassed record was established by a certain Faillos from Kroton with a 17 meter jump.

To ease the impact with the ground, athletes moved their arms forward as they left the ground. Perhaps the high jump also took advantage of the same technique to reach greater heights than athletes reach today.

There was always an oboe player at the *palaestra*. His job was not only to set the pace of exercise, but also rhythm for the launching of the discus and javelin. Discuses were made out of bronze and weighed from 1 to 4 kilograms, but children's discuses weighed less. Discuses were smeared with sand so that the fingers wouldn't slip off. Officials marked the places where the discuses fell by placing stakes in the ground as they still do today. In this way, athletes were able to test themselves against each other.

Javelin throwers are sometimes depicted with a compass in hand. This was likely to draw a circle into which the javelin had to fall. The distance that a javelin throw could cover was sometimes doubled or tripled by a type of band wrapped around the shaft and unwound as the javelin was cast, causing it to spin. The throw could also be increased by the lift applied by the athlete.

Boxers had their hands wrapped in hide. These early "gloves" went up to the forearms leaving the fingertips free, and had different shapes depending on the bout they were intended for. There were even deadly gloves with a thick leather ring held firmly in place over the

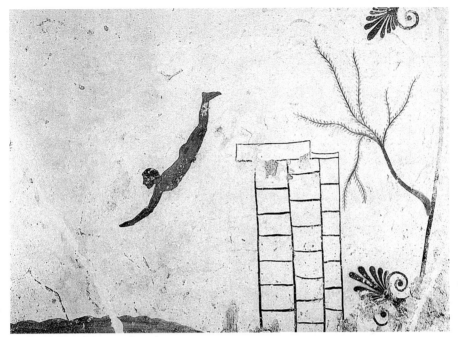

Stone slab covering in Tomb of the Diver at Paestum with the famous fresco of a man diving. In the Archeology Museum, Paestum.

knuckles by straps. One fighter named Damoxenos is remembered for having killed his opponent with one murderous blow to the belly. Gloves were also necessary for the boxing variation called *pancratio.* This was brutal and dangerous. No blows were barred, except blinding a adversary with fingers. Because the playing field had been flooded with water, it was muddy. The contest ended when one of the two muddy and blood-stained contestants raised their arm in surrender. However, the dishonor of surrender was unknown in Sparta. To avoid useless bloodbaths, other Greek cultures behaved well by not allowing the proud Spartans to participate in *pancratio.*

Unlike Athens, Rome used exercising in the *palaestra* as well as the stadium games for military training. Participation in gymnastics soon became very selective because sons of the ruling class reaped benefits in gaining the ability to become strong future combatants and commanders to keep Roman peace inside and on the frontiers of the Empire.

Gymnastics were not for everyone. It was permeated with paramilitary groups, soaked with deep political meaning and strengthened by religion to feed the warrior spirit.

Boys from Pompeii, as in other Roman cities, belonged to such groups beginning with the era of Augustus. The most politically minded youths were in sports clubs so that they could spread the principles of the new imperial ideology among the citizenry. One particular club was called *Iuventus*, the word for youth. An impressive *palaestra* was certainly built for them: 11,500 square meters with a 750 square meter swimming pool in the center that held 1350 cubic meters of water. The bottom slanted to give it a 260 centimeter depth. Ladders served as resting stops and aided getting out of the water. The pool was landscaped with trees.

In Caesar's Rome, athletic events were scarcely attended because they were considered immoral. This continued despite the fact that the Emperor Titus Flavius Domitianus (Domitian) had a splendid stadium built in the heart of the Campo Marzio, to revive the Greek sporting

Left. *Small terracotta statue of a gladiator. In the National Archeology Museum, Naples.*

Bronze gladiator helmet. In the National Archeology Museum, Naples.

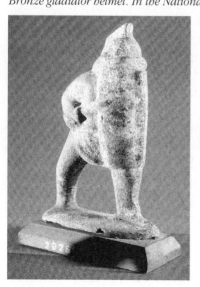
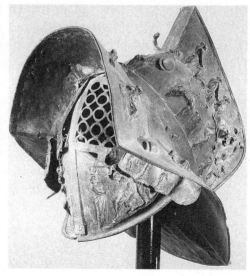

tradition. It seems that the people were used too extremely exciting spectacles and were not much attracted to those that were calmer and refined. They were drawn to gladiator contests (*gladiatoria munera*), wild beast hunts (*venationes*), bull and even rhinoceros fights, men that hunted beasts and beasts that hunted men, scenic displays from myths or history that were so real that people in the leading role always died. Nothing seemed to be too much for the people in the amphitheater. Crowds were cruelly insatiable for new and strong emotions. Seneca recounts the following:

> *Between spectacles, someone's throat is cut just to kill time.*

How could the truculent plebe, and not only, be unmoved by so much ferociousness if the Emperors themselves perpetuated the events to guarantee the celebration. Domitian is remembered for having the gymnast's interest in heart. But hadn't he distributed passes for free admission to the houses of ill repute during the games in honor of victory over the Germans? The memory of the bloody circus fight in Pompeii between the spectators from Nuceria and Pompeii in 59 A.D. must already have vanished from the minds of the spectators. It was, however, still present in the memories of some senators who prohibited gladiator contests for ten years. That was appropriate punishment, but counter productive in an Empire that used the games to keep down rebellion.

Balnea, vina, Venus corrumpunt corpora nostra, sed vitam faciunt (Baths, wines and women corrupt our bodies, but make life grand)

A Roman workday ended around noon for everyone, regardless of job and social standing. How to occupy the rest of the time until supper was a daily preoccupation for the Romans. It was especially a problem for those who did not have a comfortable home or villa. The less well off had to roam the streets or squares, promenade beneath the porticos or be left to the tediousness of doing nothing at all.

Baths were prescribed by doctors and hygienists alike. This support led the brilliant Romans to establish rules for the bath as a gateway to health and purification. Once a rich man's privilege, the bath soon became a prerogative for everyone because it was free or very cheap. This was a political move by the quick-witted Emperors to keep people from getting bored. Seeking the public good may not have been the driving force behind this preoccupation with free time. If the common people's energies were not directed, they wouldn't know how to pass away their time. Whatever the reason, the result was that innumerable people of all walks of life and both sexes went to the baths every day to reinvigorate their bodies, release stress and establish social contacts. The large bathhouses from the Imperial age looked more and more like upper-class residences, lined with iridescent marble, decorated with mural paintings and statuary. They were landscaped with gardens and parks. They even had a library. This was an excellent opportunity for citizens who would otherwise never have been able to attend a daily bath at such a low cost.

When the crowds arrived to take part in the pleasures of the baths, they were equipped with towels and ampoules containing ointments for massages. They likely passed through the entranceway of the building and went full speed down to the dressing room (*apodyterium*) hoping to find an empty cubbyhole where they could leave their clothing. Surveillance was scarce and undisturbed thieves frequently made off with garments. Patrons, therefore, had to get by on their own by taking turns at the watch, or pay someone to do it for them.

The feel of warm dry air that drew effortless sweat must have been sensational. What a stroke of intelligence to have designed and built a heating system where slow burning fire provided all the benefits, but was invisible. The elderly would still be able to recall the direct fires of their fathers, when one or more stoves were used. They must have produced suffocating clouds of smoke. In the new order, the magnificence of the Emperor was at a height. The cry of the land was: "May Jove always protect him".

The copious sweat brought on the desire to bathe, so patrons would go to the large hot tub (*calidarium*) in the middle of the room to cleanse their bodies with sodium carbonate. People would sit on the

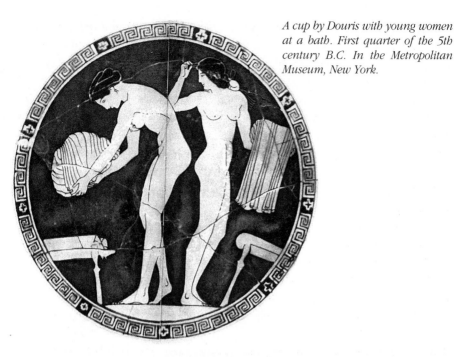

A cup by Douris with young women at a bath. First quarter of the 5th century B.C. In the Metropolitan Museum, New York.

marble steps leading into the water. Some chatted with their neighbors, others got in up to their necks to enjoy the warmth of the water that became grimy with use. It took little time, however, for the running water to return to clarity. Many felt that it was a shame that the Emperor Hadrian ordered separate baths for men and women. It was pleasing, and the daily attendance to feast ones eyes on promiscuous Roman women boosted revenues. The change was fueled by the scandal of an upper class Roman woman who frolicked around half naked, perhaps to demonstrate her absolute liberation. After this occurrence, men and women took turns at the bath. The important thing was to take advantage of every minute the setting offered.

Hot water numbs body and soul. It gives one the sensation of sweet abandonment that is hard to overcome by any method other than to douse one's self with cold water. Ancient physicians prescribed a good cold water tempering. Anyone who would prefer the Spartan bath of leaping from a hot tub to a cold one without first getting used to it was mad. Doing so was said to strengthen both mind and body. The mere thought brings on a cold chill. In the warmth of the *tepidarium*, a body would acclimatize to the room temperature until it was ready to be immersed in. The cold water tub was located in another room (*frigidarium*). On a good sunny day it was preferable to go outdoors into the garden and dive directly into the cold water pool (*natatio*). Taking advantage of the boldness of youth, boys worked backwards. They first dove into the outdoor pool or cold water *frigidarium*, then sat in the *tepidarium* to get massaged and oiled, then they took a hot bath in one of the large tubs that could hold as many as 28 people.

As expected, a crisp cool day would tend to draw people to the warmth and keep them there. While waiting to get in, there was no better place to sit than in one of the niches along the wall and take in the heat all around. The central heating worked perfectly. The *suspensurae* system was invented by C. Sergius Orata, a contemporary of Cicero who will be remembered for posterity for placing the wood stoves in the basement to heat a large zone below the pavement of the *calidarium*. The heat rose along the walls and escaped into the space created between the wall and the perforated bricks.

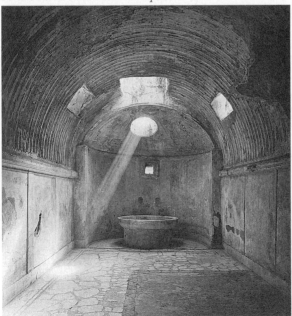

Forum baths: calidarium. Pompeii.

The large opened windows facing southwest to catch the sunlight at peak hours carried the voices and clamor of people exercising in the outdoor *palaestra*. They worked out to regain or maintain their waistline. The gymnastics in the *palaestra* next door to the baths were designed to use as many muscles as possible and get many people of all ages and both sexes to participate. Any young smirks directed at older people were strictly out of place.

One couldn't be able to blame them, however. Adults running behind large metal circles and steering them with curved metal sticks would not be inspiring. But to stay fit, the hygienists recommended that kind of exercise for the manner of running, muscle tone and balance. That game became so popular that it left the *palaestra* and was played even on the street. Quick-paced or distracted pedestrians were likely to hear the gymnast approaching by the sound of small metal rings that rolled on the ground in synchrony with the circles.

The game of triangles (*trigon*) was better at calling youth's attention. This game tested dexterity, resistance and skill, by attempting to catch as many balls as possible when thrown by another player at the corner of an imaginary triangle. The balls that were caught had to be released almost contemporarily. Servants from the baths or personal slaves picked up the balls.

Others punched a bag filled with seeds, flour and sand that hung from a rope. Imagine a brawny youth used to wrestling and *pancratio*. He wouldn't be satisfied to simply punch the *corycus* designed for weaker folk. He'd hit it hard, the contents would spill, and the game would be over for the day.

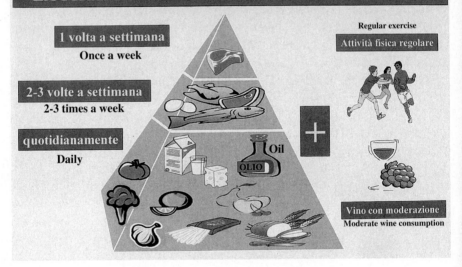

THE MEDITERRANEAN FOOD PYRAMID
LA PIRAMIDE DELLA DIETA MEDITERRANEA

1 volta a settimana
Once a week

Regular exercise
Attività fisica regolare

2-3 volte a settimana
2-3 times a week

quotidianamente
Daily

Oil
OLIO

Vino con moderazione
Moderate wine consumption

10 The food pyramid

From history to today

The association of the Mediterranean diet with some of the greatest ancient civilizations – Egyptian, Phoenician, Greek, Etruscan, and Roman – may have been coincidental, although the pioneering British nutritionist John Waterlow has argued: "It is difficult to conceive how the Greeks and Romans could have achieved such remarkable feats, which involved far more than a small elite, if they had not in general had an adequate and nourishing diet". This theory cannot be refuted by the fact that some key elements of the modern Mediterranean diet, notably tomatoes and some fruits, were introduced into the region much later; the defining elements of the diet – olive oil, grains, and wine – have been in the region for millennia.

There are several definitions of the Mediterranean diet, but in essence it emerged when poverty in the region limited access to all but locally produced plant foods. The addition of olive oil facilitated the consumption of raw or cooked vegetables, legumes, wild greens, and even cereals.

Three types of diet are widely reputed to be associated with good health and longevity, mostly on the basis of ecologic and geographic evidence: the Chinese, the Japanese, and the Mediterranean diets. Though it is not easy to compare these diets directly with respect to their healthfulness, there is good evidence that the Mediterranean diet is the realistic choice for people who engage in moderate-to-low levels of physical activity and consume moderate-to-high levels of dietary lipids. The evidence for this recommendation has been widely embraced by experts in the field.

Food geometry

The food pyramid has been developed to outline and illustrate the traditional culinary differences (traditional cuisine) continually associated with good health. These cultural models for a healthy diet are presented in the form of a pyramid to provide a general idea of the proportions of food and how often they should be eaten. It also indicates the choices of healthy foods rather than a respect for weights and measures, or daily energy allowances. The Mediterranean food pyramid serves primarily as a guideline for the public at large, especially adults, with possible and necessary modification for children, pregnant women, or people with special problems.

There is no such thing as good or bad foods. The key to healthy eating is to discover proper food balance. A balanced daily diet should be broken down into 50-70% carbohydrates (starch and sugar), 20-30% fats and the remaining 10-20% proteins. It is better to eat low on the pyramid and gradually decrease the use of foods at the top, while bearing in mind that daily calorie needs change from person to person.

The Mediterranean food pyramid provides general dietary rules that are easy to follow and get results. These recommendations are based on many studies investigating the relationship between diet and public health. With a quick sweep of the eye one may take in the entire breath of decades of scientific publications.

The base of the pyramid

Vegetable products form the cornerstone of the Mediterranean diet. Examples can be found in the typical cuisine throughout this geographic region. The North Africans serve *couscous* with legumes. Southern Europeans (Spain, Italy, and Greece) eat polenta, rice, and pasta with vegetables and legumes. The eastern regions of the Mediterranean eat *bulgur* and rice with vegetables and beans. Bread is eaten with all foods regardless of class or social standing. It is the most democratic of foods and certainly the most ancient.

Fresh vegetables, salad, fruit, seeds, nuts and olives are eaten regularly, while garlic, onions and herbs as seasonings add a touch of genuineness and strong flavor to the table. All this provides a correct supply of micronutrients (vitamins and minerals), fiber and other beneficial substances (natural antioxidants). Fresh vegetables distributed where they are picked, eaten naturally with minor culinary changes to bring out the taste, enhance this winning combination for prevention. Without considering geography, all nutritional guidelines agree on the need to eat a variety of foods. This can easily be accomplished through vegetables.

The base of the pyramid is therefore filled with foods that must be eaten on a daily basis to reap the greatest benefits. This provides a rich, varied and tasty diet that is endorsed by science. Many studies have underscored the low risk of heart disease and cancer in people who eat these foods.

Foods found in the tomb of Kha: grains, a pumpkin, a pomegranate and an egg. In the Egyptian Museum, Turin.

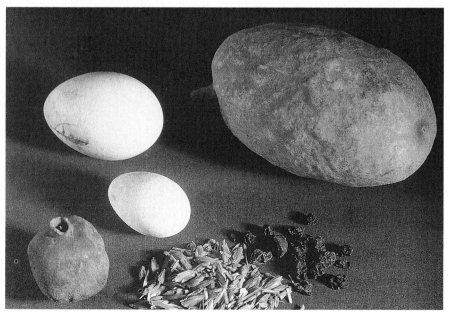

Not all carbohydrates are the same

The nutritional message that has circulated in recent years regards the ability of complex carbohydrates to promote good health. This is the same message that comes with a glance at the food pyramid, guaranteed by 6-11 portions per day of bread, cereals and grains. Complex carbohydrates are found in the starches of these foods. Simple carbohydrates (sugars) should be eaten less because their digestion and absorption raises blood glucose levels quickly after eating.

The concept of glycemic index is an important one because it tells us just how much the blood glucose will rise after introducing one food instead of another. Technically speaking, the glycemic index represents the increase in glycemia after eating a food with carbohydrates compared to the increase in glycemia caused by the ingestion of a reference food, such as bread. The higher the glycemic index for a food, the greater the blood glucose response and vice versa. The glycemic index is the expression of many components, such as the type of starch found in a food (e.g., amylose or amylopectin), the size of the food particle (whole or ground up), the presence of fiber, the degree of ripening and the way of cooking.

Some foods consistently present a low glycemic index. Compared to white bread that by definition has a glycemic index of 100, red beans have a 3-fold lower index (36). This means that the rise in blood glucose after eating 100 grams of beans will be about 3 times less than after eating 100 grams of white bread. Other foods with a low glycemic index are chickpeas (50), lentils (40), spaghetti *al dente* (45), parboiled rise (54), bran (74), toasted barley (31) and several kinds of fruit such as apples (53) and oranges (60).

The *Nurses' Health Study*, conducted on 80,000 U.S. nurses reported that a diet with a high glycemic index increases myocardial infarction. This prospective study investigated the eating habits of a large population of women over a long period of time. Another study, this time performed in the United Kingdom, observed that people habitually eating low glycemic index foods also have a favorable lipid profile. In other words, the concentration of protective cholesterol (HDL) in the bloodstream is higher than in people eating high glycemic index foods.

Although milled grain yields highly refined flour for tasty bread and pasta, it also causes a loss of important nutrients for good nutrition (vitamins, fiber and minerals). A recent study investigated the eating habits of about 35,000 menopausal American women (*Iowa Woman's Health Study*) for 10 years. A careful consideration of the women who died from coronary heart disease compared to the rest of the study population showed that eating non-refined cereals lowered the risk of coronary disease. The women who ate at least 9 por-

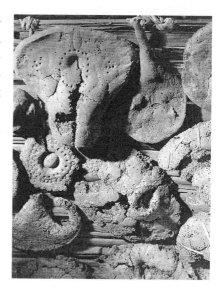

Top. *Bread from the Kha tomb at Deir-el-Medina (18th dynasty). 1567-1320 B.C. In the Egyptian Museum, Turin.*

Models of fruit and legumes found at Heliopolys, in Egypt. 2040-1640 B.C. In the Louvre, Paris.

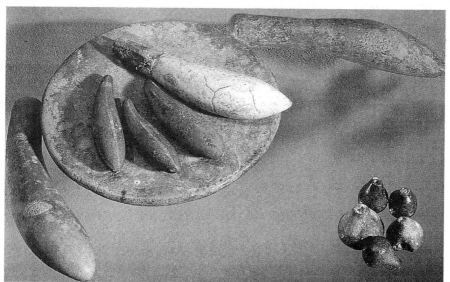

tions of unrefined cereals per week had a 30% lower risk than women eating one and a half portion per week.

There are many ways in which unrefined cereals protect the cardio-vascular system. Eating them supplies a great deal of mostly soluble fiber, folic acid, antioxidant vitamins and minerals. They also substitute for other potentially dangerous foods with a higher glycemic index, such as potatoes and white bread, or unquestionably dangerous foods like saturated fats.

A guide to proper nutrition cannot await the complete discovery of all the mechanisms at play. Scientific evidence suggests the kind of car-bohydrates to place at the bottom of the pyramid. Encouraging people to eat complex carbohydrates is simply not enough because white bread and potatoes are rapidly converted into simple sugars, and as such absorbed. Unrefined cereals ought to be the main source of car-bohydrates at the bottom of the pyramid.

Vegetarians

It has taken three years to examine 4500 studies adding up to a rich volume of 750 pages to demonstrate that cancer can be prevented even at the table. Fruit and vegetables offer the greatest protection against some kinds of tumors (mouth, pharynx, esophagus, lung, stomach, colon-rectum, but also pancreas, breast and urinary bladder). These have found their greatest endorsement in the 1997 report entitled: *Food, Nutrition and the Prevention of Cancer: A Global Perspective*, published in the United States. This monumental report claims that every year up to a quarter of a million tumors could be prevented by proper diet and lifestyle.

It has been calculated that the number of true or presumed vegetari-ans in the world number around a billion. Most are such because they are forced by poverty, religion, or environmental conditions, especially in China and India. Aside from the ambiguity brought on by the term, other factors should be taken into consideration, including the use of dairy products and the distance from the sea. People living near oceans tend to eat more fish. In the West things are not so simple. Only one or two people out of one hundred are completely vegetarian, at least in the U.S.A. Such a distinction serves to thoroughly evaluate the effects of a diet completely lacking in animal products on individual and public health.

Vegetarians belonging to the religious group called The Seventh Day Adventists eat no meat, use no spices, abstain from alcohol or coffee, and do not smoke. There is about a two million worldwide membership. The death rates compiled for some of these communities since the 1960s have now become available in California, Holland, Japan and Norway. Despite fluctuations due to confounding factors such as age and sex, deaths from cancers are from 25 to 75% lower in the Adventists than in the general population.

The situation is very much the same for other vegetarians. There was a 50% decline in tumor-associated deaths in 20,000 vegetarians living in the United Kingdom and an even lower rate of mortality in about 2000 German vegetarians. Part of the merit may be attributed to the assortment of fruit and vegetables eaten by vegetarians compared to their omnivore cousins. This choice leads to the intake of a greater amount and variety of active oligominerals from vegetables.

Ten suggestions on fruit and vegetables

1. Eating fruit and vegetables is fundamental. The minimal indispensable amount of leafy or raw vegetables is equal to the volume of a fist (knuckles down) setting squarely on the table (about 65 grams); half or three quarters of a fist for cooked vegetables. Potatoes are not considered vegetables, but an alternative to macaroni, rice or polenta.

2. Eat at least three portions of vegetables per day. The types of vegetables must change every 4-5 weeks. Increasing the portions for enhanced value is useless, but there are no contraindications.

3. Tastes change. Those who have never been fond of vegetables should be encouraged to try them again. Perhaps flavoring the dishes with herbs or cooking differently will help.

4. Minestrone, soups and sauces. These are equal to a portion of cooked vegetables when thick, and half a portion when watery.

5. Eating legumes 2-4 times a week should be encouraged. Legumes can substitute for a second course of meat, or eaten together with pasta or rice. Portions range from 6 tablespoons when legumes are fresh and 3 spoonfuls when dried.

6. Vegetables must be fresh. Vegetables in season maintain their maximum nutritional value when eaten fresh or raw. The out-of-season alternatives are frozen, freeze-dried, dried or canned vegetables.

7. Cooking. It is better to cook vegetables in water without adding salt or bullion cubes. Pressure cookers, vapor cookers and microwave ovens are acceptable. Convection ovens limit the loss of vitamins and mineral salts. Should you cook with oil, choose olive oil. Butter, dairy cream and partially skimmed milk should seldom be used. The amounts should be limited to a cube of butter, a spoonful of cream or three spoonfuls of milk.

8. Seasonings. A tablespoon of olive oil per person is enough during a meal. Two to three spoonfuls in a salad bowl for two is plenty. Go easy on salt. Toss well to better appreciate the taste of vegetables, oil and herbs.

9. Fruit. In season fruit is best. Eat no less than 2-3 pieces a day. If you cut back on bread and pasta, do not make up for it with more fruit.

10. More fruit. Consuming squeezed, centrifuged or blended fruits will enhance lose dietary fiber, minerals and vitamins. They also reduce thirst. Fruit should be eaten whole.

Milk and dairy products

Cheese and yogurt are essential ingredients for many traditional Mediterranean cuisines and contribute to the enrichment of taste as well as variety. On the contrary, milk, butter, and dairy creams are less used. Current nutritional guides suggest eating at least two or three portions of cheese per day, to receive the minimum daily allowance of calcium and high quality proteins.

It is common opinion that a high intake of calcium can reduce the risk of fractures and osteoporosis, besides guard against colon cancer and high blood pressure. To these positive considerations we must add other less desirable effects. Dairy fats are saturated. As such they are sworn enemies of arteries. Although high quality, animal proteins increase the renal loss of calcium and consequently determine a decline in the total calcium reserve in bones. Bone stores of calcium serve to balance renal excretion. It is paradoxical that a heightened risk of hip fracture has been reported in milk drinkers. What's more, populations with a low calcium diet present the lowest incidence of fractures. In Greece, for example, the risk of hip fracture almost doubled in the 1977-1987 period (from 58 cases to 97 cases per 100,000 people), in parallel with a doubled use of milk and dairy products.

The high intake of saturated fats from dairy products can cause possible damage to arteries. Similarly, a limited intake of milk, butter and cheese in the diet of Mediterranean populations may have contributed to good health. The low intake of dairy products appears to be compatible with a low incidence of bone fracture and colon cancer. Should an increase in calcium intake be required, for example in the adult population (1000-1500 milligrams/day), supplements are recommended.

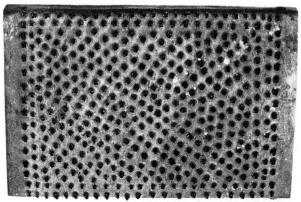

Top. *Plate with the remains of fish. Punic necropolis of Kerkauane. 5th-4th century B.C. Tunis.*

A Roman grater. In the Antiquarium of Celio.

The use of fat-free dairy products to lower fat intake without affecting calcium is certainly preferable, but may not be enough to ward off illness. The total protein intake, in fact, remains the same. We run a danger by overeating when certain that there is no fat. Finally, the missing lipids in many of these low-fat foods are generally replaced with carbohydrates. Therefore, the total energy supply is similar to the original product.

As for public health, the low-fat or fat-free industry is an important one, but harmful to school aged children and low socioeconomic levels of the population, as well as for the people living in developing countries that receive surplus fat as a humanitarian aid. Cheese and butter are questionable assistance packages. Countries in East Europe have long benefited from surplus butter from the European Economic Community. The result has been a doubling of cases of coronary heart disease since 1960.

The diets eaten in Mediterranean countries typically contain large amounts of vegetables and fewer dairy products from goats, sheep, cows, water buffaloes and camels. There is reason to believe that eating even fewer dairy products may be better for health. On the other hand, fresh or fermented cheeses whether soft or hard, and yogurt contribute substantially to the pleasantness of the Mediterranean diet. So, small portions of fermented dairy products play a fundamental role in this culinary tradition. Grating some high fat cheese, such as "parmigiano" (parmesan) is a clear example of an approach that incorporates this product in a healthy food plan that is also very gratifying to the taste.

Fats and oils

One problem nagged the epidemiologists who studied the eating habits of the Mediterranean countries. How could they explain places such as Crete, where people enjoyed an excellent state of health despite their intake of fats that made up about 40% of the daily energetic requirement? A high fat diet was also typical of Finland with the highest rate of coronary heart disease. It appears, therefore, that besides quantity, quality of fats in the diet plays a pivoting role. The unifying feature of most Mediterranean populations is the broad use of olive oil as a main source of fat. This substitutes for the saturated animal fats so typical in northern European cuisine.

Saturated fats and dietary cholesterol tend to increase the levels of blood cholesterol, the polyunsaturated vegetable oils and fish oils tend to lower cholesterol, while the monounsaturated oils (olive oil) are neutral. Thinking only in terms of total cholesterol circulating through the bloodstream may be misleading. We now know that there are different kinds of cholesterol, some can be harmful to arteries (the low-density lipoproteins [LDL] for instance), others are protective. The high-density lipoproteins (HDL) make up a small part of total cholesterol, about 20%, but are inversely correlated with coronary heart disease. In other words, the higher the HDL, the lower the risk of heart disease. Expressing the concept with the total cholesterol/HDL ratio, the lower the ratio the lower the risk. Decreasing total cholesterol and/or increasing HDL will have that effect. This occurs whenever the intake of monounsaturated or polyunsaturated fats is great and when saturated fat intake is low.

All fats by nature tend to increase cholesterol and thus HDL, except polyunsaturated hydrogenated oils contained in some vegetable margarines. Such fats are termed "trans", perhaps because they are masked by innocuous agents.

A good supply of monounsaturated and polyunsaturated fats appears to be crucial for a correct diet. Olive oil is rich in monounsaturated fatty acids (oleic acid) and less rich in polyunsaturated fatty acids, especially the omega-3 fatty acids. An alternative source of protective omega-3 may be found in fish, or some vegetables (rapeseed, linseed, soybean, and nuts).

Vegetable oils supply important tocopherol for the diet. Olive oil contains approximately 12 milligrams of alpha-tocopherol (vitamin E) for every 100 grams of oil. The union between a diet rich in monounsaturated fats and discrete amounts of vitamin E may protect against atherosclerosis.

Although several studies suggested that the substitution of saturated fats in the diet with polyunsaturated fats could prevent vascular disease, no study had ever evaluated the effect of a Mediterranean diet on the incidence of heart disease. It took the French in the *Lyon Diet Heart*

Study to compare the cardiovascular effects of two different diets in subjects who had had a myocardial infarction. The experimental group with 302 subjects followed a typical Mediterranean diet with a percentage of total fat less than 35%, saturated fat less than 10%, monounsaturated fat more than 10%, linoleic acid (omega-6) less than 4% and linolenic acid (omega-3) more than 0.6%, with a omega-6/omega-3 ratio of about 5.

The following six dietary commandments were given to the experimental group:

- more bread
- more vegetables and legumes
- more fish
- less red meat (beef, pork, horse) and more poultry
- never a day without fruit
- no butter and creams, a special margarine instead.

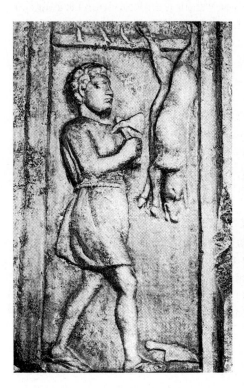

Butchering a pig. A relief from Aquileia. In the Museo Civico, Verona.

A shepard milking a goat. A relief from the Imperial age. In the Museum of Roman Civilization, Rome.

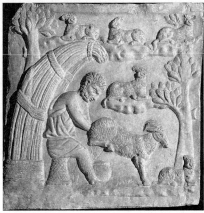

Because a Mediterranean diet had to be by definition rich in monounsaturated fatty acids, the French investigators had to face the problem of forcing ample amounts of olive oil (an average of 25 grams per
day) on that population of countrymen. The winning move was to
choose rapeseed oil, with the same characteristics as olive oil, and
present it as margarine. So the French got their spread. At the end of
only two months, the mortality curve between the two groups began to
fork. The group treated with the Mediterranean diet had fewer deaths
than the group on standard diet (more polyunsaturated omega-6 oils
coupled with a traditional post-infarction diet). Forty-six months after
the study began, the Mediterranean diet reduced mortality by 70%.

To lower cholesterol, the diet in Western society is based mainly on
polyunsaturated fatty acids instead of saturated fats. A polyunsaturated
fatty acid such as linoleic acid found in corn and sunflower oils is thus
recommended. Linoleic acid has 18 carbon atoms (C18), with two double bonds (2n) and belongs to the omega-6 series (18:2n-6). But linoleic acid can have undesired side effects. It favors the oxidation of LDL
that promotes atherosclerosis and increases platelet aggregation.
Linolenic acid, on the other hand, belongs to the omega-3 series of fatty acids (18:3n-3) and is plentiful in rapeseed, soybean, linseed and
dried nuts. It is interesting to note that the two populations with the
longest life spans, the people from the island of Crete and the Japanese
from the island of Kohama, seem to eat the most linolenic acid.

The *Lyon Diet Heart Study* provided us with the first demonstration
that a Mediterranean diet, such as that eaten on Crete, although adapted to a western population, protects the heart more than a standard
post-infarction diet. A lower intake of saturated fats, a higher intake of
oleic acid (found in olive and rapeseed oils), natural antioxidants (occurring in fruit and vegetables) and linolenic acid, associated with little
meat and wine, are very likely winning combinations. They show that a
global approach to eating is worth more than a single choice. The findings are even more impressive when we consider that the French already have one of the lowest cardiovascular disease rates in the world.
For men it is second only to the Japanese.

It is hoped that a diet with the same characteristics as that used in
the French study can be used elsewhere and not only in the popula-

tions with a high risk of heart disease. Roughly 50% of the people living in Western countries are destined to die of heart disease, especially heart attack. Since most people ignore their destiny, it would be wise to instill preventive eating habits.

Meat and fish

Epidemiological investigations carried out on populations living in Western countries indicate that an excessive intake of red meat, veal, pork, lamb, is associated with an increased incidence of chronic and degenerative diseases including heart disease and some cancers (colon, perhaps prostate, and others). The most consistent evidence for this association is provided by the comparison of disease rates between Seventh Day Adventists who eat meat rarely or not at all and non vegetarians, who eat meat every day. The latter have a 60% greater likelihood of dying from coronary heart disease.

It is still unclear whether it is the fat in meat to solicit these harmful effects. Carcinogens could form during cooking, especially by grilling, cooking over a flame, or frying. Nitrosamines, suspected source of all our troubles, were first identified in burned meat and can induce tumors in laboratory animals. It seems, however, that these substances are not responsible for tumors in humans. Hence, the mechanisms that underlie carcinogen-mediated tumor initiation after a rich meat diet remain a mystery.

Meat contains little fiber and has no natural antioxidants. Eating meat on a daily basis means that you eat fewer vegetables, which are rich in antioxidants. Red meat is also the leading source of methionine in the diet. This amino acid is the direct metabolic precursor of homocysteine, another amino acid, which does not become a building block of protein, but is harmful to arteries. It is plausible, though not demonstrated, that a high intake of meat can raise levels of homocysteine in the bloodstream. The toxic effects of homocysteine and the ways to prevent them will be covered later in another chapter of this book.

Bearing this in mind, the guidelines established by the American Department of Agriculture just a few years ago are unconvincing. These guidelines recommend eating 140-196 grams of meat per day in a healthy diet.

Traditionally, Mediterranean populations eat little meat and have fewer health risks, but most important of all, have individual and public health profiles that are far better than those found in industrialized nations that eat more meat.

The amount of fish eaten in Mediterranean countries varies. The Spanish, the Portuguese and the inhabitants of Corfú eat the most. The people living in South Italy and Crete eat the least fish. Such a finding should in theory suggest a marginal role for fish in the Mediterranean diet. However, clinical studies disprove this view.

The eating habits for a large group of American male physicians (almost 20,000) were followed in a 12-year study. Those who ate fish at least once a week presented a risk of sudden death 30-40% lower than those who ate fish less than once a month. The fatty acids in fish also belong to the omega-3 series (like linolenic acid), but the names are more complicated. Eicosapentaenoic acid for instance has twenty carbons and five double bonds giving it a formula of 20:5n-3, and docosaesaenoic acid has twenty-two carbon atoms and six double bonds (22:6n-3). It is likely that these fatty acids replace linoleic acid (omega-6) in the lipid bilayer of the cell membrane, stabilizing changes in cardiac rhythm that may be fatal (sudden death).

Principles for eating well: the thirteen commandments

1. Diet and eating
   a) Eat a balanced diet that is varied and based on vegetable matter.
   b) Favor a diet rich in fruit, vegetables and non refined starchy food.

2. Body weight
   a) Body mass index (weight in kilograms divided by height in square meters) in adults must be kept on the average between 21 and 24, considering 18.5 and 25 as the lower and upper limits, respectively.

b) Avoid losing or gaining weight beyond the average values and try not to increase more than 5 kilograms during adulthood.

3. Physical fitness

a) Be physically active and adopt an active lifestyle.

b) Should your job increase a sedentary lifestyle, take a daily walk for about an hour or take up an activity equal to at least one hour of gymnastics per week that uses the whole body.

4. Fruit & vegetables

a) Make vegetables at least 7% of your dietary calories.

b) Eat 400-800 grams or five portions of fruit and vegetables per day all year long.

5. Other vegetable foods

a) Include foods that are rich in proteins, starch (better when unrefined) until you cover 45-60% of calories eaten. Refined sugar must not exceed 10% of your calories.

b) Eat 600-800 grams or at least seven portions a day of assorted cereals, legumes, tubers, roots. They are best when milled the least. Limit the amount of unrefined sugar.

6. Alcoholic beverages

a) No alcohol is advisable and every excess must be avoided. For those who are used to drinking, 5% of the calories for men and 2.5% for women are enough.

b) Up to two glasses of wine a day for men, and one glass of wine for women at mealtime is permissible.

7. Meat

a) The amount of protein coming from red meat must not exceed 10% of the total protein in the diet.

b) If you do not intend to give up red meat, the total contribution of calories should not exceed 80 grams per day. Chicken or game or fish is a better choice.

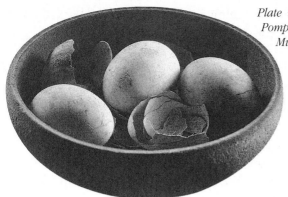

Plate with the remains of eggs from Pompeii. In the National Archeology Museum, Naples.

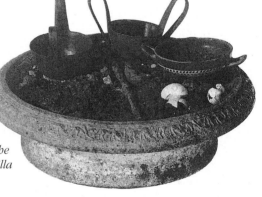

Burner with the remains of funeral meal from Cerveteri. Second half of the 6th century B.C. In the Museum of Villa Giulia, Rome.

8. Fats & oils

a) The total fatty acids must assure a supply of calories between 15 and 30% of the total calorie intake.

b) Limit the use of fatty foods, especially those containing animal fats. Season with vegetable oil, above all with olive oil.

9. Salt

a) The total amount of salt for an adult must not exceed 6 grams per day.

b) Restrict salt in cooking, eating salty foods and table salt. Use herbs to flavor fresh foods.

10. Preserving

a) Save perishable foods in such a way as to limit fungal growth as much as possible. If you are not planning to eat something right away, refrigerate or freeze it.

b) Never eat foods left for extended periods at room temperature. They can become contaminated with micotoxins. Whenever food is not eaten within a few days, freeze it according to supplier recommendations.

11. Additives

a) Establish the maximum acceptable values and check to see whether safety levels have been respected for preservatives, pesticides and other chemical contaminants.

b) When contents are within safety levels, preservatives, additives and other residues in food and drink are not dangerous. Exceeding the established levels may be risky to health, especially in developing nations.

12. Preparation

a) It is advisable to cook meat or fish at low temperature.

b) Avoid burning sauces. Fish and meat grilled directly over an open fire and smoked meats should only be eaten occasionally.

13. Dietary supplements

a) A balanced diet is sufficiently protective and does not require food additives.

b) Follow these recommendations and supplements should be unnecessary.

Fundamental principles for a correct diet (a) and dietary advice (b), beginning at age two.

11 Health benefits of the Mediterranean diet

A word from science

Modern scientific research has revealed the benefits of the Mediterranean diet. Not only does it provide the natural elements to live a healthier life, but combined with exercise it can also influence life expectancy.

Diet is a cornerstone of cardiovascular disease prevention and treatment efforts. At the core of dietary guidance are the recommendations to decrease saturated fat and cholesterol and to consume more fruit, vegetables, and whole grain products. Information from an extensive database, especially regarding saturated fat, indicates that these diets significantly lower blood cholesterol level, a major risk factor for cardiovascular disease. Consequently, it is beyond debate that these diets reduce cardiovascular disease risk.

Nutritionists have sought to develop effective implementation strategies, including identifying dietary patterns that augment the beneficial effects of these diets. The provocative evidence from the Lyon Diet Heart Study suggests that a Mediterranean-style diet (emphasizing more bread, more root vegetables, and green vegetables, more fish, less beef, lamb and pork replaced with poultry, no day without fruit, and butter and cream replaced with oleic acid and more α-linolenic acid) has effects that may be superior to those observed for the usual diets recommended for cardiovascular prevention.

Radicals, better bound than free

Never as in the last years of the second millennium has life expectancy at birth been so high. This is evident for Western cultures, but is also to a lesser degree true for developing countries. A sharp decline in the infant mortality rate that occurred following large scale vaccination and the availability of medicines has played a major role. The world's population is aging. Affluent societies are aging more than economically unstable ones and the rich more than the poor, everywhere. The need to meet the medical challenge of the elderly is leading biomedical research into avenues that investigate the aging process and associated diseases such as diabetes, atherosclerosis and hypertension.

Much attention has been paid in recent years to free radicals as mediators of biological aging. The reverberations from this research have been great, not only in scientific journals, but also by the mass media. Television bombards us with commercials advertising a series of products that claim to regenerate the body by reducing free radicals. Are free radicals truly enemies of public health, or are they scapegoats?

First, it would be a good idea to determine the extent of the problem and the risks for public health, especially nutrition. Free radicals are by definition unstable molecules because they contain one or more unbalanced electrons in their outer orbital. What does this mean for the lay-person? In normal atoms the orbitals are spaces where electrons are likely to be found around a nucleus of protons and neutrons. Orbitals normally contain an even number of electrons, and thus have no apparent electromagnetic energy, they are stable. This helps to explain why these molecules with outer orbits containing one electron alone behave like small magnets. They are strongly reactive and tend to react chemically with any substance that can donate an electron to form a stable orbital. In other words, a molecule defends itself from unwanted reactivity by searching for stability. This occurs at the expense of a free radical itself, when it fills its orbitals and becomes stable. The disappearance of an intruder free radical may occur in various ways, but mainly by pairing the uneven electron with a similar one from another radical, or transferring an electron to other molecules.

How and why are free radicals formed? In virtue of their extreme reactivity, free radicals have very brief biological life spans on the order of thousandths or millionths of a second. This makes tracking their destiny by scientific instrumentation difficult. Free radicals are produced by ionizing radiation, ultraviolet rays, environmental toxins (cigarette smoke, exhaust fumes, hepatotoxic drugs, and chemotherapy), food toxins, ethyl alcohol, medicines such as paracetamol and antimalarial agents.

Bear in mind that the branch of life from which human stems uses oxygen for cellular respiration. Paradoxically, the characteristics of oxygen such as its ubiquity and hunger for electrons renders the metabolic pathway chosen by mother nature for the survival of aerobic organisms (living in the presence of oxygen) a source of oxygen radicals.

The toxicity of these radicals is linked to their ability to bring about a change in the molecule and alter its function within an organism. A typical example is the damage caused to nucleic acids that store an organism's genetic information. Free radical-damaged genetic material will likely cause mutations, denaturing of membrane proteins with consequent changes made to membrane transport, or finally, loss of enzyme function so needed by an organism for its chemical reactions.

Let us not attribute all of our woes to free radicals. Some of their effects are beneficial and indeed required for cell survival. The mechanism by which leukocytes (white blood cells) scavenge for bacteria at the site of an infection, called phagocytosis, makes use of free radicals produced on a large scale to eliminate the microorganisms. Free radicals also serve in the synthesis of vital substances for the organism, such as cerebral neurotransmitters and thyroid hormones, to name just a few.

The concept of oxidative-stress should be understood as the balance between production of free radicals and their elimination. Whenever the production exceeds the elimination, the slight damage over the long term can accelerate aging. Fortunately, mother nature has interceded to provide organisms with a series of defenses – the antioxidants. Not all antioxidants that protect us from risks are known. Actually, most remain to be discovered. These defense systems are very complex and often interact as an antioxidant network. Antioxidants may be enzymatic and non enzymatic (enzymes increase the rate and yield of a reaction), intracellular or extracellular, hydrosoluble (soluble in water) or liposoluble (soluble in oil). For example, superoxide-dismutase is an enzyme the catalyzes (accelerates) the reaction that produces hydrogen peroxide (H_2O_2) from two molecules of an oxygen free radical, the superoxide anion radi-

cal (•O$_2^-$). The negative sign
indicates that the molecule is
electrically negative and that
there is only one electron in
its outermost orbital. In turn,
the hydrogen peroxide will be
cleaved into water (H$_2$O) by
yet another enzyme, termed
catalase. Some free radicals
are neutralized in such a way.

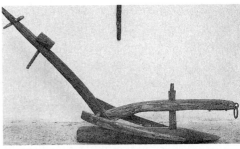

An ancient wooden plow is a silent testimony to the hard life lead by farmers.

Glutathione is a non enzymatic substance that serves as cofactor (a
non protein substance required by an enzyme for activity) in many reactions that degrade radicals. Since glutathione is a free radical scavenger,
its maintenance in a reduced chemical state (GSH) is necessary (when
reduced it gains electrons). In other words, when scavenging as a radical, glutathione oxidizes by losing electrons. In the process it passes
from the reduced state (GSH) to the oxidized state (GSSG) which is no
longer a scavenger. Other substances, some of which are enzymes,
recharge GSSG by converting it to its original reduced form so that it
can go about its important role. The protection afforded by antioxidants
derives from their involvement in radical scavenging reactions that yield
non reactive radicals. These are almost inert, or anyway rechargeable.

Vitamin E is a non enzymatic liposoluble antioxidant contained in
most vegetable foods. There is major storage of this vitamin in cell membranes since they are almost
entirely made up of phospho-
lipids. When behaving as an
antioxidant, vitamin E destroys
radicals by donating electrons,
but at the same time becomes
oxidized. In doing so the molecule becomes inactive against
other radicals. Such "suicide"
inhibition occurs for the common good. Vitamin C (ascorbic
acid), however, comes to its

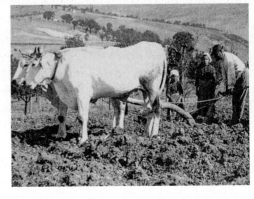

Farming life with a team of oxen pulling a plow.

rescue by assuming the oxidized element of the vitamin E molecule thus regenerating it for future use. In turn, ascorbic acid is cleaved to dehydroascorbic acid and restored to its original form by other molecules. This chain reaction of mutual assistance for an antioxidant gives us insight into the complex system of degrading waste molecules produced during normal cellular activity.

Antioxidants, the natural ones are better

Some eating habits can increase oxidative stress in the following two ways: by suddenly increasing the production of free radicals that overwhelm defensive mechanisms and by introducing few natural antioxidants in the diet that help organ systems. Such diets may contain excessive calories, be lacking in essential amino acids (the building blocks of proteins), or have an insufficient number of vitamins or oligoelements involved in antioxidant enzymic reactions. Copper and zink are oligoelements required by the superoxide-dismutase enzyme to function correctly.

It is commonly believed that atherosclerosis is associated with aging and deterioration of higher brain function. Atherosclerosis concerns the structural integrity of an artery and is considered a typical disease of wellbeing and a public health threat. The damage that it causes to the heart (myocardial infarction), the brain (stroke), the kidneys (renal failure) and peripheral circulation (gangrene) is the major cause of illness and death in Western countries. The rest of the world is tending in this direction. World Health Organization (WHO) figures attest this worldwide catastrophe and warns that cardiovascular disease will be the leading debilitating illness in just twenty years. Together with cancer, cardiovascular disease is the leading cause of death.

In the past, human disease was mostly the result of microbial infection; today it is hinged on the formation of radicals (especially atherosclerosis and cancer). Free radical-induced changes in the gene make up is a plausible explanation for the relationship between oxidative stress and tumors. The hypothesis that oxidative changes in some lipid components of the blood trigger and maintain atherosclerosis is supported by evidence.

Principal natural antioxidants

	Mechanism	Where found
Carotenoids	Antioxidant	Vegetables and citrus fruits
α-β carotene		Carrots,
Lycopene		Tomatoes
Lutein		Spinach
Zeaxanthin		
Ascorbic acid	Antioxidant	Citrus fruits, tomatoes, potatoes, leafy vegetables
Tocopherols	Antioxidant	Wheat germ, oat flour, nuts, vegetable oils
Phenols	Antioxidant	Fruit and vegerables, tea, red wine
Flavanols		
Flavones		
Anthocyanins		
Catechins		
Proanthocyanidins		
Tannins		
Allyl sulfide	Regenerate reduced glutathion (GSH)	Garlic, onions, leeks
Limonoids and tiocyanates	Form protective enzymes	Citrus fruits, chicory
Monoterpens	Antioxidant	Carrots, broccoli, cabbage, eggplant, peppercorns
Xanthophylls	Block the oxidation of fats	

Fat is not usually soluble in water. To be transported in blood (mostly water) lipids require carrier proteins. These are denominated lipoproteins (fats and proteins) whose role is to orchestrate fat distribution through the bloodstream. Some of these substances such as low density lipoproteins (LDL) carry cholesterol. When in excess, cholesterol is considered harmful for arteries. However, it is not as much the amount of LDL in the bloodstream that is damaging as the amount that deposits below the endothelium (the thin membrane lining the inner walls of the blood vessels). For a series of reasons that can be ascribed to the scarce antioxidant capacity of the microenvironment below the endothelium, LDL gets oxidized by free radicals. Such a process changes their shape enough not to be recognized by the cells designated to digest them (macrophages). These devour them uncontrollably, as if they were foreign molecules to be destroyed. This continuous accumulation results in the inability of the macrophages to digest them. These macrophages become transformed into foam cells which by definition compose the first atherosclerotic lesion known as a lipid strip.

Support for the free radical hypothesis to explain the pathogenesis of the two greatest public health threats (atherosclerosis and cancer) has come from several epidemiologic studies carried out on large segments of the population. Findings reveal that foods, such as cereals, fruit, vegetables and vegetable oils, high in natural antioxidants, are associated with a lower risk of disease. This evidence has been strong enough to persuade several scientific organizations such as the American Heart Association, the American Cancer Society, and above all the American Department of Agriculture to establish guidelines for food hygiene that incorporate a high percentage of vegetable products.

The protective role of vegetables against cancer and heart disease is likely the result of their composition. Many nutritional substances within these foods still remain to be characterized. It is also probable that the right combination of many factors come together when a varied diet of vegetables is eaten. Let us not forget that there is no cure-all that can ward off and prevent illness. Unfortunately, we don't know yet what composition, percentage and dosages of the likely blend of compounds, will confer protection.

The initial enthusiasm for antioxidant therapy to prevent or treat cardiovascular disease has been substantially tempered by a series of negative clinical trials for both vitamin E and vitamin C, and beta-carotene. Given the lack of proved efficacy of antioxidants in clinical trials to date, antioxidant vitamin combinations above the recommended dietary allowances should not be recommended for prevention or tratment of cardiovascular disease. More importantly, the use of antioxidants could be hazardous, especially in combination with lipid-lowering drugs. The next chapter in the antioxidant saga will depend, at least in part, on the results of ongoing clinical trials.

Diet and cancer

Cancer generally has a complex etiology with multiple risk factors that involve an interplay between genetic and environmental influences. Geographic differences, trends over time in risk of cancer, and detailed studies of migrant populations overwhelmingly implicate environmental exposures as major causal factors and often identify the responsible carcinogens (tobacco, alcohol, radiation, occupational toxins, diet, drugs). From an arrey of studies has come the widely accepted estimate that 80 to 90 percent of human cancer is due to environmental factors. Yet, in the past 15 years, the explosion of molecular genetic has overshadowed environmental explanations by revealing genetic mechanisms underlying cancer. This is why the current confusion about environmental and genetic risk factors for cancer is not surprising.

The most accurate assessment of an individual's risk for developing cancer would be an estimate of dietary and other environmental exposures (*nurture*) as well as information on interindividual differences in genetic susceptibility (*nature*). Links between dietary factors and genetic susceptibility are being investigated through studies in human twin pairs.

Comparisons of the concordance of cancer between monozygotic and dizygotic pairs of twins provide information on whether the familial pattern is due to hereditary or environmental influences. If concordance for cancer is higher among monozygotic twins (who share all genes) than among dizygotic twins (who, on average, share 50 percent of their segregating genes), genetic effects are likely to be important. If, however, the concordance is similar for both types of twins, then shared environmental factors are probably important. A recent study included more than 10,000 cancers in a total population of nearly 90,000 twins in Scandinavia and provided valuable information for the nature-versus-nurture debate. In general, environmental factors were the dominant determinats of the site-specific risk of cancer: for stomach, colorectal, breast, and lung cancer, estimates of proportion of risk due to environmental effects run 65 percent or greater. For cancer at the common sites in monozygotic twins, the rate of concordance was generally less than 15 percent. Thus, the fatalism of the general public about the inevitability of genetic effects should be easily dispelled.

Diet is one of the most important lifestyle factors and has been estimated to account for up to 80 percent of cancers of the large bowel, breast and prostate. Even lung cancer may have a dietary component, although cigarette smoking is the overwhelming cause of this and contributes also to other cancers (oropharyngeal, oesophageal, bladder). Evidence from epidemiologic and corroborating experimental studies strongly supports relationships between dietary constituents and cancer risk, suggesting that, in general, vegetables, and fruits, dietary fiber, and certain micronutrients appear to protect against cancer, whereas fat, excessive calories and alcohol seems to increase cancer risk. Other environmental characteristics, for example, degree of physical activity and obesity, also are lifestyle factors that appear to have major influences on cancer risk.

How nutrients can modulate the risk of cancer

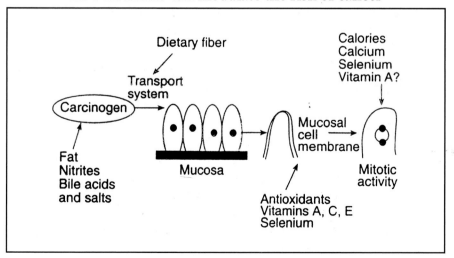

Cancer is a multi-step process involving a cancer producing agent (carcinogen) which must reach a cell, pass through its membrane, and exert its influence, usually when the cell is undergoing mitosis.

- *The nutrient itself is a carcinogen or leads to the formation of carcinogens.*

Fat probably leads to the formation of carcinogens by two mechanisms: breakdown of fat by intestinal bacteria to products that are carcinogens; increased secretion of bile secondary to a high fat diet.

- *The nutrient is involved in transporting a carcinogen to a susceptible cell.*

Dietary fiber, particularly insoluble fiber, increases intestinal mobility and reduces transit time through the colon. Hence, any carcinogen is excreted more rapidly and is in contact with mucosal cells for a shorter time.

- *The nutrient affects the permeability of the cell membrane to a carcinogen.*

Antioxidant vitamins may protect cell membrane from leaking and therebe being penetrated by carcinogens.

- *The nutrient affects the rate of mitosis or cell division.*

Calories are necessary for cell division. Reduced caloric intake would protect against cancer by reducing the number of mitosis in the colonic or ductile mucosa and thereby reducing the overall time when cells would be susceptible to the action of any carcinogenic agent.

The cancer inhibitory effects reported for plant foods may be attributed partly to a variety of antioxidant constituents, including β-carotene, vitamin E, vitamin C, selenium, and certain phytochemicals (polyphenolics, carotenoids). It is likely, however, that numerous compounds contribute to the overall protective affect. The encouraging epidemiologic evidence prompted controlled clinical trials, the only definite way to test the hypothesis that chemopreventive agents, including dietary antioxidants and phytochemicals, can reduce cancer risk. In general, the results of such intervention studies carried out in Western cultures, which tend to be well nourished and not deficient in multiple micronutrients, have been disappointing, specially for β-carotene: the Physicians' Health Study found no evidence of benefit, while both the Alpha-Tocopherol, Beta-carotene Lung Cancer (ATBC) Prevention Trial, and the Beta-carotene and Retinol Efficacy Trial (CARET), carried out in populations at high risk of lung cancer, found evidence of harm with β-carotene (16% and 28% higher incidence of lung cancer, respectively). Moreover, three recent clinical trials provide no evidence that a diet low in fat and high in fiber, high-fiber cereal supplement, or calcium supplementation reduce the risk of recurrent colorectal adenomas. There may be many reasons to eat a fiber-rich diet: the soluble fibers help maintain normal blood levels of glucose and cholesterol, considered risk factors for cardiovascular disease. However, preventing colorectal adenomas, at least for the first three to four years, is not one reason.

The existence of an association between diet and nutrition and cancer risk is not in question. At present, there is no evidence that isolated supplements of vitamins or antioxidants help to prevent cancer. A diet high in fruit, vegetables and whole grains, and low in meat, fat, and salt, but containing adequate minerals and vitamins, is a good prophylactic for preventing many chronic diseases of lifestyle. Further, a plant based food economy is much more sustainable than one based on livestock. Providing that other lifestyle factors are also taken into account, the diet for cancer prevention can, on the basis of current knowledge, form the basis for a rational public health policy.

Homocysteine: the revolution

There is a growing body of clinical and experimental evidence indicating a direct correlation between homocysteine in the bloodstream and cardiovascular disease. Homocysteine is crucial in the metabolism (a two-step process of building and breaking down molecules in the body) of sulfur-containing amino acids.

The most interesting results have come from the Nurses' Health Study, begun in 1980 on 80,000 American nurses aged between 30 and 55 years, and followed-up for 14 years. Data regarding eating habits were gathered by mail questionnaire. The study considered the intake of folic acid and vitamin B6 in the diet, as well as that supplied by multivitamin complex tablets. The risk of fatal and non fatal acute myocardial ischemic events (infarction, angina) was significantly less in subjects in whom folates and vitamin B6 intake were high. The protection was high regardless of whether folic acid and vitamin B6 came from the diet or from supplements.

A table set with a plate, a flask and a pitcher. Perhaps even the Italian painter Morandi could not have done any better.

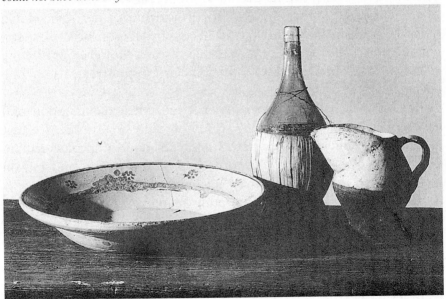

In the case of folic acid, the decrease in risk derives from the reduction in homocysteine levels, accelerating its transformation in methionine, an amino acid precursor of homocysteine. The more folic acid and vitamin B6 introduced, the lower homocysteine levels become. The lowest risk is obtained when the daily folic acid and vitamin B6 exceed the recommended daily allowances. This occurs when folates exceed 400 micrograms per day and the amount of vitamin B6 is more than 3 milligrams per day. To modify homocysteine levels at least 400 micrograms of folates per day are needed.

An elevated blood level of homocysteine in the blood can harm the blood vessels by increasing the risk of thrombosis in arterial vessels: the platelets adhere to each other and to the inner lining of the vessels (endothelium), the cells of the endothelium decrease their ability to produce substances that dilate the blood vessels, and clotting occurs. Levels of homocysteine can be sharply increased in the bloodstream by feeding a person methionine which changes to homocysteine in the body. The test calls for the administration of 0.1 gram of methionine for every kilogram of body weight. For instance, a 70 kg adult would assume 7 grams of methionine in 200 milliliters of fruit juice. When this test was used on healthy volunteers it was seen that homocysteine levels rose from two to three-fold within four hours. At the same time, endothelium loses some of its ability to protect the blood vessels and becomes more susceptible to insult.

More space ought to be given in the diet to foods containing substances that can lower blood levels of homocysteine. Yeast, spinach, asparagus, tossed salad, salmon, liver, dried figs, black berries, dried fruit and hazelnuts are all rich in vitamin B6, B12 and folic acid. These micronutrients can reach body tissues after eating fresh fruit and minimally cooked vegetables.

To receive enough folates to prevent a rise in homocysteine, cereal flours could be enriched. This is simple to do, inexpensive and enormously advantageous for health. To date no deleterious effects from high doses have been reported. Folic acid and B complex vitamin supplements are necessary whenever the diet is not able to supply necessary amounts.

There is an ocean of difference between just picked and refrigeration for several days, particularly where vegetables are concerned. A remarkable fluctuation in the amounts of nutrients, such as vitamins and antioxidants occurs. Freezing works better than refrigeration in maintaining antioxidant properties as close as possible to freshly picked foods. After a week of refrigeration at 4°C, vegetables lose about 26% of their ascorbic acid (vitamin C); freezing on the other hand, causes a 15% loss. This was true in research carried out on thirteen commonly eaten vegetables such as spinach, green peas, potatoes, carrots and parsley.

The recommendation to eat fresh vegetables refers to in-season produce that has been adequately stored. Otherwise, frozen vegetables are preferable to greenhouse vegetables. Because greenhouse plants grow too quickly, are supplied with all the water they need in a temperature-controlled environment and treated for pests, they have minimal antioxidants. Vegetables picked when ripe and rapidly frozen, on the other hand, retain their antioxidants.

Does wine make good blood?

Is wine healthy or does it harm the coronary arteries? We are obliged to ask this question because excessive alcohol has long been known to damage the liver, affect childhood growth, pregnancy, and old age. The main cause of alcohol toxicity likely derives from its change into acetaldehyde by the alcohol-dehydrogenase enzyme. A surplus of acetaldehyde causes a drop in the liver stores of reduced glutathione, an important antioxidant. This is why alcohol-induced liver disease is seen as a free radical disturbance.

For some years the international scientific community has been faced with the need to address a concerned public about some paradoxes that have emerged from the literature. A paradox is by definition a phenomenon beyond explanation, or something that goes against what is known and accepted. The best known nutritional contradiction fed to the public by the mass media during a much followed television broadcast is "the French paradox". Morley Safer coined this expression in a 1991 broadcast when commenting on the findings from a World Health Organization-sponsored study named MONICA (MONItoring CArdiovascular diseases) that revealed a paradox. How could the inhabitants of Toulose, France, have a mortality rate for chronic disease far lower (more than 50% less) than the Americans (Stanford) or the British (Glasgow) with matching plasma cholesterol levels, arterial blood pressure and exposure to smoke? The paradox became even more intriguing with evidence that the French generally eat more meat and more fat than other populations in the Mediterranean Sea. In theory this should have enhanced the atherosclerotic process instead of slowing it down.

It has long been known that people living around the Mediterranean Sea have a much lower mortality rate for coronary heart disease than people in Northern Europe. Having a cholesterol level of 225 milligrams per deciliter of blood in Naples, Italy, is quite another thing than having it in Helsinki, Finland. In other words, the same risk factor damage the arteries less in Naples than in Helsinki. The chance that people living in the sunny territories around the *Mare Nostrum* have protective factors inherent to the lifestyle and cuisine has created the myth of the Mediterranean diet.

Suspect naturally fell on wine consumption since France is a leading producer. An examination of the literature on the topic led to the conclusion, in 1993, that a moderate alcohol consumption protects against heart disease. More recent epidemiological studies carried out on many people, such as the 22,000 American physicians, or the 86,000 American nurses with an even longer follow-up of twelve years, confirmed a more favorable mortality profile for the light drinker.

Should one drink hard alcohol or wine? If there were a good balance it would be enough to indicate the amount of alcohol that could be drunk each day that is not harmful and then use it in several foods. If the recommended allowance is 30 grams of straight alcohol, it would be the same as drinking hard drinks (60 milliliters - 50% proof), beer (2 cans - 5% proof), or wine (300 milliliters - 10% proof). There is reason to believe, however, that wine is a better choice. Wine is a complex water-based alcoholic drink made from fermented grape juice. Wine contains as much as 5 grams of natural antioxidant polyphenols per liter. The antioxidant strength of these substances are greater than antioxidants such as vitamin E.

The polyphenols are a heterogeneous group of antioxidants and research has shown them to be complex; there are several flavonoids in wine such as anthocyanidins, catechins, flavones, flavanols and anthocyanins. Concentrations of flavonoids range from 1-3 grams per liter of wine. The flavonoids are pigmented derivatives of the grape skins and, to a lesser extent, the seeds. Thus, red wine made by fermenting the mash over an extended period of time is rich in polyphenols. Flavonoids have been known for some time to protect the hearts of tea drinkers and lower plasma cholesterol (especially proanthocyanidins) by sparing vitamin C.

Recently, other antioxidants have come to light such as resveratrol, a rather peculiar phenol compound. Resveratrol seems to behave like a phytoalexin. This is an allelopathic compound which plants produce when subjected to stress or under attack by parasites, especially the funguses *Botrydis cinerea* and *Plasmopara viticola*. A 50-100 microgram per gram concentration of resveratrol is found in grapes, while from 1.5 to 3 milligrams per liter may be found in red wine.

It is interesting to note that outside of wine, peanuts and mulberries, nothing else we eat contains resveratrol. Why have researchers focused more of their attention on this particular compound than investigating flavonoids, as well as the other 500 or more oligoelements found in wine? The answer comes again from history and research. Traditional Chinese and Japanese medicine has always employed medicinal herbs. The traditional medicine named *Kojo-Kon*, used to treat a range of disorders, among which atherosclerosis, contains resveratrol. Research has shown this substance to be a strong antioxidant, at least as strong as the flavonoids epicatechins and quercetin. Moreover, experimental evidence performed on laboratory animals has shown that resveratrol protects against tumors enough to warrant further investigation as a human anticancer agent.

The French paradox could be explained by the "time lag" hypothesis. According to this intriguing hypothesis, the lower cardiovascular mortality in France (about a quarter of that in Britain) results from the

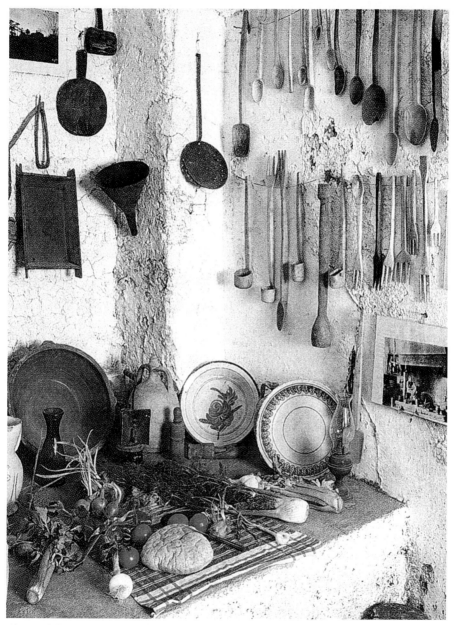

The work bench of an old Mediterranean kitchen, when the white washed background set off the colors of vegetables.

lower animal fat consumption and serum cholesterol levels the French men had before 1970. Such a time (20-30 years) was needed to obtain the present low mortality rate from ischemic heart disease in France. If the French paradox will in time dissolve is uncertain; the Mediterranean diet hopefully will remain.

Wine is a true phytocomplex in which the compound effects exceed those of the single parts. Even Hippocrates said:

Wine is an extraordinarily appropriate thing for man, if the proper amount is administered during health and illness according to body build.

Paracelsus many centuries later said:

Everything is toxic, nothing is toxic, everything is in the dose.

Finally, more recently Pasteur informed us that:

Taken in moderate amounts, wine is the healthiest and most hygienic drink.

Oleum, ad antiquo

Olive oil is relatively low in saturated and high in monounsaturated fats. It also contains a good amount of vitamin E. Although consumers who used it for centuries were unaware, these features have made olive oil the true prince of the Mediterranean diet. The distinctive characteristics of its lipid content make olive oil preferable not only to other oils, but to other vegetable oils and even to complex carbohydrates. Obviously, all these considerations are not based on the findings of better health conditions in populations that regularly use olive oil, but derive from many epidemiological and clinical investigations performed over the last ten years which have placed olive oil in its proper perspective in the scientific community.

Even compared to other vegetable oils considered harmless because they are rich in polyunsaturated fats, the monounsaturated oils (among which olive oil) are less able to cause oxidative damage to low density lipoprotein (LDL). This process of LDL oxidation is held to be exceedingly important as it sets off changes in the arterial walls of the coronary arteries, thus increasing the risk pathology. Olive oil has been the principal source of dietary fat for millennia without causing such public health threat. The use of other vegetable oils rich in polyunsaturated fats is too recent to draw conclusions on their safety over long-term use.

Olive oil also has one up on carbohydrates. A diet that is rich in monounsaturated fatty acids is better at increasing plasma levels of High Density Lipoproteins (HDL) than one with many complex carbohydrates (bread and pasta). Unlike LDL, the HDL category of lipoproteins protect the coronary arteries.

There is, however, a basic problem that must be considered in the relationship between the various components of the Mediterranean diet. Because olive oil improves taste, more vegetables and legumes around the Mediterranean Sea are eaten. For many people it would be unthinkable to eat these amounts of vegetables without the taste and consistency of olive oil. This happy union between vegetables and olive oil has made culinary history and principles of education in which taste and health go hand in hand.

This beneficial strength of nature seems to hold its own against dietary rules that limit the total consumption of fats to no more than 30% of total calories taken in. The diet eaten by the inhabitants of Crete in the 1960s contained 40% fats, but at that time coronary heart disease was 90% lower than in the United States and the prevalence of breast tumors in women was roughly half.

But not all the Mediterranean peoples eat so much fat. A good example of this variety may be found in the diet eaten by the inhabitants of southern Italy at the time of Key's report. Then, the daily fat intake was 28%. This also suggests the existence of more than one healthy Mediterranean diet model. One of these variants could be the diet eaten in the past by the southern Italians, with relatively low total fat, moderate use of olive oil, fruit and vegetables, and plenty of grain cereals. Another variant was eaten by the Greeks. This featured a considerably higher fat intake coming from olive oil, much fruit and vegetables and a moderate intake of grain cereals.

What has changed since then? In light of the prevailing western eating habits, can diet models from the regions examined still be considered protective for health? Previously, butter was seldom used in food preparation, while margarine was completely unknown. The use of both these foods has been on the rise for the last 30 years, as has other vegetable oils cheaper than olive oil. These and other changes in the eating habits have contributed to the increase in risk factors for chronic disease among Mediterranean populations; for example, higher blood levels of cholesterol, increased incidence of hypertension and obesity. Obviously this has led to an increased incidence of cardiovascular disease, diabetes and some kinds of cancer correlated to improper dietary habits.

Italy is seen by others as a cornerstone of the Mediterranean diet. Its wealth in foods and culinary styles have set trends and passed beyond the Alps. But there is a paradox; Italy is changing. In the twenty years from 1965 to 1985, the intake of bread within the adult population examined fell from 350 grams per day to 194 grams per day, whereas

Left. *The small stove with the lid burned charcoal or nutshells to help farmers through the winter.*

An old hutch: a mouse trap can be seen to dissuade daring rodents.

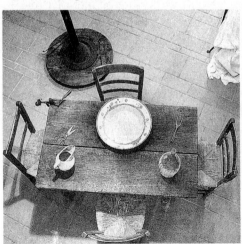

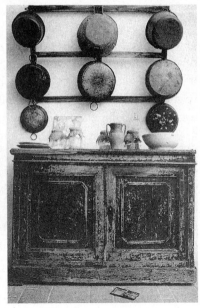

olive oil at 30 grams per day is threatened by foods offering less consistent lipid profiles such as meat, milk and dairy products. These increased by 300%. In the ten years between 1981 and 1991, the consumption of beef and cheese had a major increase (+8% for animal fats and +6% for animal proteins) luckily counterbalanced by the increased intake of legumes and vegetables (+30% vegetable proteins), fruit, fish, vegetable oils (+18%), and the drop in use of butter, eggs, refined sugar and liquor.

Despite the changes in diet, the Mediterranean countries still appear to be favored. The protective role of the myriad vegetable compounds present in fresh produce, wine, olive oil, and in whole grain cereals could hold the key. Despite the recent changes in Mediterranean eating habits linked to several different factors such as fads, culture, declining tendency to share a meal around the table with the family, little time to cook, and quick meals, the cardiovascular health profile of Mediterranean countries is still better than the rest of Europe.

More tea, please

Tea drinkers consuming at least four cups of the fragrant drink each day have a lower risk of dying from ischemic heart disease, better known as heart attack. This finding has emerged from recent epidemiological studies that have focused attention once again on the benefits of a diet based on natural products. One study in particular is worthy of attention because it was conducted in Holland. The Netherlands are not typically linked to the Mediterranean diet and this supports the possible globalization of a safe diet.

Eight hundred and five citizens at Zutphen, between the ages of 65 and 84 years, were followed for five years. State of health, eating habits, flavonoid and natural polyphenol intake, were recorded. The following compounds with the most antioxidant strength were considered: flavanols, quercetin, kaempferol, myricetin, the flavones apigenin and luteolin. Within five years after the study's onset, forty-three subjects had died from heart attack. Each of the deceased had declared an intake of dietary flavonoids lower than the subjects still alive. In other words, the intake of flavonoids corresponding to a mean of 26 mg per day, as much as in four cups of tea, protects against myocadial infarction. What if one drinks less than four cups of tea? Have no fear. There is equal protection from onions and apples. The greatest sources of flavonoids in the study were divided among tea (61%), onions (13%), and apples (10%).

As for the intake of other vegetable products, tea drinkers generally eat more fruit, vegetables and carbohydrates, use fewer fats, drinks little coffee and smoke less. To avoid false hopes, it must be underscored that people with a low vascular risk generally lead a healthy lifestyle. Drinking a cup of tea each day, but continuing to eat unhealthily is wrong, and in the end can be dangerous because it denies the real problem of choosing a proper lifestyle.

From across the Atlantic comes more good news for tea drinkers. A study carried out on three hundred and four people of both sexes living in Boston who had had a heart attack and the same number of healthy people revealed that the risk of coronary heart disease was inversely proportional to the daily drinking of tea. The risk was cut in half in the people that drank one or more cups of tea each day compared to those who drank no tea at all. It was also found that drinking coffee did not increase the risk of heart disease.

The health virtues from habitual tea drinking likely derive from the high flavonoid content in tea. Flavonoids are potent antioxidants that block lipoprotein LDL oxidation and thus ward off potential harm to the arteries. Other mechanisms can also play a role. Platelets are cell fragments that circulate in the bloodstream and stop hemorrhages. However, platelets can be dangerous should they act on a mature atherosclerotic plaque, because they can contribute to vessel occlusion leading to infarction or stroke. Modern medicine is now able to downregulate and inhibit the ability of platelets to aggregate and form a network upon which a thrombus is built. This can prevent cardiovascular events. It seems that the flavonoids are even able to inhibit platelet aggregation, thus contributing to their protective effect on the heart and vessels.

Researchers from Stockholm have recently demonstrated that a substance contained in green tea is able to block the proliferation of blood vessels in laboratory animals. The ability to block angiogenesis opens avenues of research on possible cures of diseases expressing new blood vessel growth, such as tumors and blindness associated with diabetic retinopathy.

People should be cautious in their choices. Not all teas are alike, at least regarding their amount of catechins. Black decaffeinated tea contains less, whereas herb tea contains none at all. It is important for tea producers to determine just how much of these substances are contained in their products and the best way to avoid losing them during preparation.

Another look at menopause

Women tend to live longer than men. With the continual rise in life expectancy, women undergo a roller-coaster relationship with their ovaries. Today at the start of the new millennium, we must consider that as women live to be eighty years old and over, their fertile life adds up to 35-40 years. This is less than their non fertile life span, seen as the sum of the post-menopausal and pre-menstrual periods.

The problems menopausal women encounter are essentially due to the missing estrogens supplied by the ovaries. Estrogens are a class of hormones that distinguish the fertile period, and that stop being produced by the ovaries sometime around age fifty. This event causes a series of more or less unpleasant reactions, such as hot flashes, headaches, sleeplessness, mood change, as well as a series of metabolic changes that can seriously compromise health. Osteoporosis is a major skeletal threat that predisposes the spine to collapse, leads to progressive shortening in stature in the elderly, and femur or hip fracture. The rise of blood lipids, especially triglycerides and cholesterol, is a strong risk factor for the cardiovascular system. Weight gain due to a slowed basal metabolism causes adipose tissue to accumulate in the abdomen and in the upper regions of the body. Menopausal women tend to lose the usual gynoid pattern of fat deposition (in the hips and thighs) and gain a masculine fat build up along the waist.

Phytoestrogens, which are diphenolic compounds derived from plants and converted into estrogenic substances in the gastrointestinal tract, are being increasingly promoted as the "natural" alternative to estrogen-replacement therapy. Like other plant substances, phytoestrogens have their maximum protective effect when taken directly with natural foods and not as supplements. Phytoestrogens are found in three hundred different plants, not all of which are edible. A large number, however, remain to be chosen according to personal taste. Their names are not easy to remember: genistein, daidzein, enterolactone, enterodiol, uquol. Whether one remembers their names or not, these substances belong to three large families, the isoflavones, the lignans and the coumestans. Such a distinction serves to identify the foods which contain them.

Isoflavones are found in soy products. Soybeans are the richest, while other derivatives such as soy sauce, flour, ground up plants, milk and oil contain less. For anyone who dislikes the taste of soy, it can be substituted with Mediterranean whole grain cereals and legumes (lentils, beans and peas). In this case as well, attention must be made to the different ways these foods are handled. Whole grain cereals such as wheat, barley, rice, rye and oats contain higher amounts isoflavones than the same refined cereals. As with all replacement therapies, the estrogenic strength of this substance can vary from woman to woman even with the same amounts of food. This influences the phytoestrogen level in the bloodstream.

The other group of phytoestrogens occurs in foods that are more in tune with the Mediterranean eating habits, such as fruit and vegetables, oil made from olive seeds, beer made from hops and grain whiskey. But first place goes to leafy vegetables, colored fruit and linseed oil. The coumestans are mostly found in sprouts.

Epidemiological observations have revealed that Asiatic populations have a lower incidence of cardiovascular disease and hormone-dependent tumors (breast, endometrium and colon). Studies carried out on Japanese women have demonstrated, for example, that not only is the risk of breast cancer inversely related to soy use, but tumors, should they appear, are less invasive, less aggressive and produce fewer lymph node metastases. As for endometrial cancer, if the incidence in the United States is twenty-five cases out of a hundred thousand, in Japan or in Singapore the incidence is only two cases out of every one hundred thousand. Ethnic background has little to do with it, because the Chinese and Japanese immigrants in North America lose their protection in one generation.

Until data are made available from controlled studies on the benefits as well as dangers of phytoestrogen supplementation, a more "natural" alternative may be the consumption of six to eight portions of fruit, vegetables or legumes a day.

Exercise and poor habits

The small town of Framingham, a few miles from Boston, is famous the world over for a study that took place there fifty years ago. Epidemiologists from Harvard had the far-sighted idea of following citizens over a period of time to determine the rate of fatal and non fatal cardiovascular events and their causes. The scientific community owes much to the *Framingham Heart Study*. The concept of coronary risk factors is just one reason why. This grew out of the investigations that shed light on causes inducing coronary heart disease (CHD), such as hypertension, cigarette smoking, high cholesterol levels and even diabetes.

Some fifty years later, the *Framingham Heart Study* is still cited. A new analysis of data shows that half of men and roughly a third of women less than forty years old are destined to develop CHD at sometime in their lives. Should these findings be confirmed by other epidemiological investigations and above all if they are valid for all countries, there will be immediate practical and worrisome implications. Generally, people increase their health efforts at around age fifty, without realizing that damage begins very early, even though the disease develops in later years.

The social impact of cardiovascular disease in Western countries is devastating. One out of every two men will have problems associated with atherosclerosis of the coronary arteries. It is a paradox that despite the strong evidence, this problem falls on deaf ears, while people are more inclined to overestimate the risk of cancer. And yet a fifty year old woman has a three-fold higher chance of developing CHD than breast cancer.

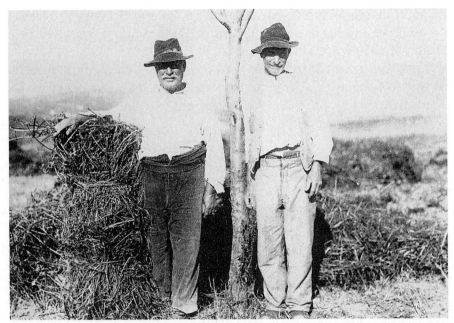

It is difficult to determine when this picture was taken and where these two peaceful farmers come from: farming life is universal.

The strong message that has emerged is that young adults and the elderly must change their lifestyles because coronary heart disease does not just affect the middle aged. Changing lifestyles is an important strategy to prevent CHD, but whether it could change the course of disease had not been demonstrated until researchers from California working on the *Lifestyle Heart Project*, a study of three hundred patients with severe coronary stenosis requiring revascularization (bypass or angioplasty). One hundred and ninety-four patients in the study group were prohibited from smoking and prescribed an intensive program including a controlled average diet of 1850 calories (less than what single individuals previously ate) and a high intake of vegetable fats (10%). The following major food categories were represented: fruit, whole grain cereals, vegetables, soybeans, legumes, skimmed milk. The treated subjects were also trained to do physical activity, such as walking an hour per day, or, provided that they were physically fit, to do a light work out in the gym. In addition, they were instructed on how to keep daily stress under control with psychological support.

After five years, those in the treated group, unlike the controls, were all thinner, had toned muscles, good blood pressure and remarkably lower cholesterol levels. Compared to the control group that followed the usual rules to prevent cardiovascular disease and in whom there was a progression of coronary atherosclerosis, the experimental group experienced a 4.5% reduction in coronary narrowing after one year and 7.9% after five years. This obviously was responsible for a 50% drop in the number of heart attacks, and the avoidance of revascularization in one hundred and fifty of the one hundred and ninety-four patients in the study. Finally, the treated group had a drastic reduction in the number of angina episodes compared to the initial values. There were 91% fewer episodes after one year and 72% fewer after five years. None of the patients required medication to lower cholesterol.

There is no doubt that a global approach based on modified lifestyle and not just one risk factor, is more likely to improve an already existing atherosclerosis. But for those who are unable to get themselves organized, aiming at less is still important. Visiting China one is mesmerized by people performing unusual movements out in the open air. The movements are enchanting gesticulations and pauses that involve most of the muscles of the body. *Tai chi* is a common exercise of the elderly, but also has a young following. A group of researchers from Baltimore has demonstrated that *Tai chi* may be classified as a light exercise that can lower arterial blood pressure in the same way that heavier aerobic exercise can.

The elderly are usually reluctant to do even light physical activity. Even taking a walk may generate insecurity because of fears of traffic and delinquency. Just the same, everyone should practice some physical activity. The choice of exercise is personal, but even light exercise done regularly is healthy.

Three years of smoking causes a 50% increase in a typical atherosclerotic lesion, such as that seen on the carotid artery by ultrasound. It takes three years for the carotid artery to thicken by 27 microns (a thousandth of a millimeter) in non-smokers and 41 microns in smokers. The relative limitation of these data must not let the important observation become overshadowed. It has in fact been shown that for every 163 micron increase in thickness of the carotid wall, the risk of cardiovascular events almost doubles (43%).

However, even non-smokers exposed to passive smoke are at risk. This may be measured in a roughly 5-7 micron increase in the thickness of the carotid wall compared to a non-smoker or ex-smoker who is not exposed to passive smoke. The ex-smokers are more at risk than people who have never smoked. The progression of atherosclerosis seems to be correlated with the number of cigarettes smoked. It is well to underscore the fact that both active and passive smoke damages the heart by subjecting the endothelium and plasma lipids to free radical stress. In each breath of smoke there are about one hundred billion molecules of free radicals that impose a remarkable antioxidant workload on the body. No one is surprised therefore to learn that a smoker's lungs have lower levels of vitamin E, which is used up in the battle against smoke, and that the membranes of red blood cells have a reduced capacity to sweep away free radicals.

Can diabetes be prevented by changes in lifestyle?

Type 2 diabetes mellitus, previously known as non-insulin-dependent or adult-onset, accounts for 75-90% of cases of diabetes, depending upon the ethnic background. Type 2 diabetes has previously been erroneously referred to as *mild diabetes,* because it is often asymptomatic in terms of the classic symptoms of diabetes such as thirst and polyuria. However, it should be referred to as a *silent killer,* where cardiovascular disease is the principal cause of death for about 70% of type 2 diabetic patients.

The World Health Organisation has predicted that the global prevalence of type 2 diabetes will more than double from 135 million in 1995 to 300 million in 2025. The regions with the greatest potential increase are Asia and Africa, where type 2 diabetes could become two to three times more common than it is today. It is felt that lifestyle changes, with diets high in saturated fat and decreased physical activity, together with an increased longevity, are the main factors in this explosion of type 2 diabetes.

Type 2 diabetes results from the interaction between a genetic predisposition and behavioural and environmental risk factors. Although the genetic basis of type 2 diabetes has yet to be identified, there is strong evidence that such modifiable risk factors as obesity and physical inactivity are the main nongenetic determinants of the disease. For centuries, fatter and sedentary people have been considered more likely to get diabetes. This thought has been confirmed by recent studies indicating that weight loss and exercise improve the biological action of insulin at target tissues and also increase insulin secretion from the endocrine pancreas.

The Finnish Diabetes Prevention Study examined the effect of changes in lifestyle on the development of type 2 diabetes in high-risk subjects. All subjects had impaired glucose tolerance – an intermediate stage in the natural history of type 2 diabetes characterized by a lesser degree of hyperglycemia. Impaired glucose tolerance is associated with an annual rate of progression to diabetes of 1 to 10 percent. A total of 523 overweight subjects with impaired glucose tolerance were randomly assigned to either a control group, which received general information on changes in lifestyle, or an intervention group. Subjects (265) in the intervention group met a nutritionist seven times during the first year and every three months thereafter; the visits were designed to encourage specific changes in their lifestyle. Goals for changes were established in five categories: a reduction in weight (by 5 percent or more), a reduction in fat intake (to less than 30 percent of energy intake), a reduction in saturated fat intake (to less than 10 percent of energy intake), an increase in fiber intake (to at least 15 grams per 1000 calories each day), and an increase in exercise (to at least 30 minutes per day). After 4 years, the risk of developing diabetes was 58 percent lower in the intervention group (11%) as compared with the control group (23%). The reduction of diabetes was highest in the group with the largest changes in lifestyle.

Other studies paid close attention to the role of dietary composition in diabetes incidence. In the Iowa Women's Health Study, 35,988 women, aged 55-69 years, free of diabetes, were followed for 11 years. Intake of fat was assessed from a validated food-frequency questionnaire. The results show that substituting polyunsaturated fatty acid intake for saturated fatty acid was inversely associated with diabetes risk: the consumption of vegetable fat was associated with a 22% reduction in new cases of diabetes in the highest consumers (median 41.7 grams per day). This study can well compared with the most recent results from the Nurses' Health Study which followed a cohort of younger women (34-59 years) for 14 years: a similar inverse association between diabetes risk and intake of vegetable fat was observed. The results of these recent epidemiological studies support the evidence that vegetable fat may reduce the risk of type 2 diabetes, at least in women. However, the general picture is that intake of saturated fatty acids and their associated dietary variables, dietary cholesterol, meat intake, and animal fat, are associated with increased risk of diabetes.

The current guidelines of the American Hospital Association place increased recognition on the diet as a whole rather than on single nutrients. This is a laudable approach from a health education as well as a public health point of view and relates to the prevention of diabetes. Indeed, the adoption of a Western (Anglo) diet may increase the risk of diabetes in Pima Indians. Compared with the Indian diet, the Anglo diet consists of less complex carbohydrates, dietary fiber, and vegetable proteins, and presumably less vegetable fat. Moderate energy intake (relative to the level of physical activity), increased intake of dietary fiber (soluble as well as nonsoluble), and a reduced intake of saturated fat, partly replaced by starch and vegetable fats (polyunsaturated as well as monounsaturated fatty acid), are the dietary recommendations that best describe the most recent findings. Importantly, these suggestions are in agreement with recommendations on the prevention of other chronic diseases, such as heart disease.

At present, the results of these studies should encourage physicians and other health care providers to persevere in the difficult task of promoting a healthy lifestyle, since by doing so they will give patients a better chance at a life less burdened by many diseases.

Nutriceuticals, what are they?

Nutriceuticals are gaining importance and will continue to do so with their diffusion by the mass media. The birth of a new word is an important occasion, especially when there are economic interests at stake. The term "nutriceuticals" does not escape this unwritten rule and indicates a series of products that will surely make an impact. They are sold over-the-counter and used to promote good health. As usual, it is likely that physicians will know less than the well-read consumer of non academic magazines that insist upon the benefits of these substances, whether real or not.

Despite the varied interpretations and linguistic variations, the term has been coined to describe products that contain natural elements, such as vitamins, amino acids and herbs that have been shown by clinical

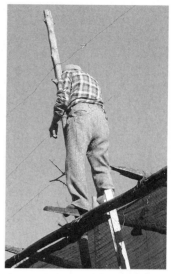

Top. *This adventurous old man still has good balance as he ties the wires for grapevines.*

Cleaning salt tubs: salt extraction by evaporating seawater is as old as time.

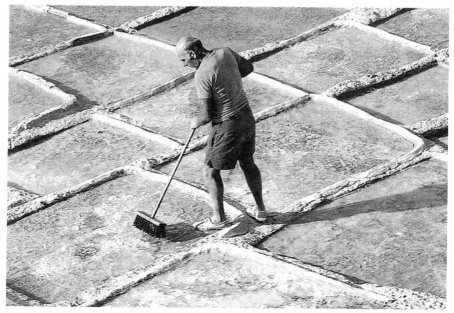

studies to be useful. The federal Food and Drug Administration has given no official statement regarding nutriceuticals, because many of these elements belong to accepted categories such as medicines, dietary supplements, health foods and food additives.

Aside from the vitamins that already have a consolidated market, some of these products are advertized to improve heart performance and make the heart healthy.

Coenzyme Q10 is a soluble antioxidant in lipids that helps vitamin E to regenerate when depleted by attacking free radicals. The proposed action mechanism for coenzyme Q10 is inhibition of lipoprotein LDL oxidation and damage to the inner lining of the arteries. The molecule is quite well known, but clinical findings are too few to prescribe it as other heart medicines.

Lycopene is a carotenoid responsible for the red color of tomatoes. It is a strong antioxidant. Lycopene may even be more potent than beta-carotene and responsible for the protective cardiovascular effects originally attributed to that molecule. In one study (EURAMIC), high tissue levels of lycopene were associated with a lower risk of myocardial infarction. The substance even seems to possess a protective role versus carcinomas of the prostate and gastrointestinal tract.

There are four thousand or more natural flavonoids in fruit, vegetables, red wine and tea. They are responsible for the color, the taste and consistency of these natural products. The interesting health properties of flavonoids have already been described. However, something more can be said.

Genistein is found in relatively high amounts in soybean sprouts. This substance inhibits the formation of thrombi by effectively retarding the processes that lead to closure of atherosclerotic vessels.

Quercetin is the most common flavonoid in food. Among its beneficial effects are inhibition of platelet aggregation and oxidative changes in LDL.

The aqueous extract of *Vaccinium myrtillis* is rich in antioxidant substances and prevents oxidation of LDL. The antioxidative potency even seems to exceed that of vitamin C.

Chinese liquorice (*Glycyrrhia glabra*) has been used for more than 6000 years in medicine. Its cardioprotective activity is linked to its antioxidant, antiplatelet, anti-inflammatory and antiviral effects. Eating too much, however, may cause a rise in arterial blood pressure in susceptible people.

Finally, there is L-arginine, an amino acid endowed with rather peculiar characteristics. L-arginine is a precursor of nitric oxide, which received so much attention from the scientific community and the 1998 Nobel Prize for Medicine for its discoverers (Furchgott, Ignarro, Murad). This molecule is normally produced by the endothelium and is the strongest vasodilator known. The stretching that the arterial walls undergo from blood flow is enough to release nitric oxide. This in turn regulates the artery wall tension moment by moment. The effects of nitric oxide as an antiatherosclerotic agent is more interesting. This is mainly attributed to its ability to sweep away free radicals, especially the superoxide anion radical which is so harmful to blood vessels. The coronary dilation brought about by nitroglycerin (used in medicine for almost a century) is due to its change into nitric oxide once in the body. Dietary supplements of L-arginine must be seen as increasing the natural stores of nitric oxide.

The potential value of nutriceuticals in treating heart disease must not be underestimated. On the other hand, it is hoped that these substances will undergo the test of rigorous clinical studies before being prescribed routinely.

A lesson from centenarians

The number of elderly reaching one hundred years of age is on the rise. It is estimated that there are a hundred thousand very old individuals in the world today. Just forty years ago, there were an emaciated group of ten thousand. They are the subject of curiosity and jealousy. How can one live to be one hundred, at least how have these people managed to do so?

First of all, it is necessary to discard old beliefs. The belief that living longer means having more illness is turning out to be wrong. At least 30% of the interviewees living to the ripe old age of one hundred have intact cognitive faculties. Their brains are clear and present minimal pathologic changes. Of the three thousand eight hundred and fifty-three century old men who met in France in 1990, clinical findings were collected on 700 cases. Fifty-eight percent were in such a state of health that researchers took no hesitation in defining as good or very good.

According to a common conviction, the demographic increase in the number of people living to be one hundred depends on intensive medical care which has lowered mortality rate in the very old. Broken hips, for example, are a plague to the elderly, but these can be treated quickly enough followed by a return to daily activities. Some thirty years ago the management was conservative, but most people died from venous thrombosis that formed during immobilization and the embolism which followed. Cataract surgery has granted elderly individuals the continuance of a satisfying lifestyle. Vaccines protect against flu epidemics. Treating high blood pressure and other risk factors lowers the sickness and deaths from heart disease.

But there must be something else besides improved medical care. Frenchmen living beyond one hundred years are described as calm, communicative, optimistic and tolerant. Their Swedish counterparts are more responsible, skillful and less apt to attacks of anxiety. Americans on the other hand seem to handle stress better than others who do not live to be one hundred. Since personality is relatively uniform throughout adult life, it is presumable that these features in the elderly help manage adversity and perhaps lengthen life.

At any latitude and under any climate, centenarians are those who have eaten moderately and done physical activity during their lives.

What lessons can one learn from the lifestyles of people reaching one hundred years? Certainly not how to live to be one hundred, at least not yet. One can learn how to use their years better. It would be ideal to live most of ones life in a state of good health. Utopia? Perhaps not, if one thinks of the many participants in the *New England Centenarian Study* who were in good physical shape in their ninth decade of life.

The slogan "active aging" was coined on April 7th 1999 (World Health Day), but the effort is projected into the new millennium. Stay in good physical and mental health while getting old has been promoted by the WHO as an imperative to the world. The message is directed both to industrialized nations that for some time have been addressing the needs of an aging population and to developing nations undergoing demographic explosion. Growing old in a healthy way begins at birth and all ages should therefore try to achieve good health.

There are no lifestyle changes, surgical procedures, vitamins, antioxidants, hormones, or techniques of genetic engineering available today with the capacity to repeat the gains in life expectancy that were achieved during the 20th century. If there is going to be another quantum leap in life expectancy at birth (20 to 30 years or more), these large gains will have to come from adding decades of life to the lives of people who reach the ages of 70 and older. Modifying endogenous biological processes to achieve this goal, although theoretically possible, will be much harder than reducing children's death rates from infectious and parasitic diseases.

True prevention begins by applying what we already know: eat right, exercise, avoid being overweight, abstain from smoking, and be screened for common diseases. All this may be translated into a longer and healthier life. There is no single thing that one can do to live longer and healthier. It is wise to be aware of individual risk factors, face them, and change what can be changed. Take care of yourself. That is the only hope to increase survival.

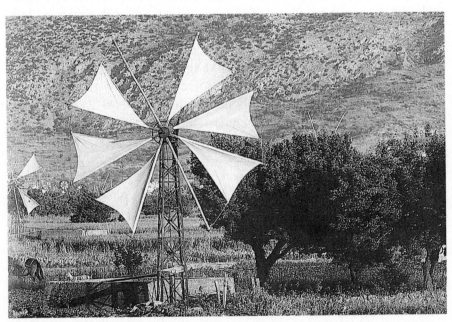

Windmills on the high central planes of Crete.

12 Health and diet

The triumph of taste and color

The diet eaten by the Mediterranean populations has precious historical, cultural, and culinary value. To safeguard the "Mediterranean factor" that has continued to play a fundamental role in combating numerous diseases, it is necessary to rediscover the pleasures of a healthy diet and remember its blessings on health. The Mediterranean diet is both tasty and healthy. Such a combination is often elusive when it comes to eating and health.

The pioneering studies of Ancel Key and Flaminio Fidanza have allowed us to rediscover and see the healthy diet eaten by the historical populations around the Mediterranean Sea, passed down since the 10th century B.C. These eating habits offer an important key to understanding the people, their civilization and history.

The lands bathed by the *mare nostrum* offer delights that express eating and gastronomic traditions in taste, smell and color that are difficult to match. The Mediterranean diet is rich, well balanced with cereals, vegetables, blue fish, fruit, monounsaturated and polyunsaturated fats, lean meat, eggs, cheeses and wines. The foundation of the "Mediterranean diet pyramid" consists of cereals (pasta, bread, rice and other grain products), fruits and vegetables. Since they are at the bottom of the pyramid, they outweigh other foods on higher levels. As one progresses to the top, the mass lessens.

Cereals, vegetables, fruit, and olive oil make up the bulk of the Mediterranean diet, whereas dairy products and red meat are used sparingly. Because dairy products and meat contain saturated fats, they tend to raise blood cholesterol levels.

Fish is an important food. Since prehistoric times fishing has provided populations living along the Mediterranean shoreline with significant stores of food. As the centuries passed, artists glorified fishing. Fishermen, boats and fish became iconographic material for engravings and ceramics. The high quality proteins, containing many essential amino acids, and iodine in fish are merited with safeguarding Mediterranean peoples from thyroid disease.

Aside from the pleasure that it adds to eating, wine in moderation protects the circulatory system.

The Mediterranean diet is a triumph of colors and tastes that consolidate cultural traditions. It strongly represents the imagination of the civilizations that have inhabited this geographic area.

Diet and health

The study by Ancel Key entitled *How to Eat Well and Stay Well: The Mediterranean Way*, demonstrated that foods eaten by people living on the shores of the Mediterranean Sea help prevent heart disease and some tumors. Because it is well balanced, the Mediterranean diet guarantees a better quality of life, a positive attitude and protection against several illnesses.

In April 1997 an International Consensus Statement was made by a group of leaders in the field of human nutrition. Based upon available evidence of health benefits derived from eating traditional Mediterranean foods, this diet was promoted as a cultural model for all European countries.

Fruit, **vegetables** and **legumes** provide dietary fiber, important minerals such as selenium, vitamin E and vitamin C, antioxidant carotenoids, and other natural biologically active substances. Vegetables have been shown to have an anticancer effect for several types of tumors, especially those of the digestive tract and those linked to hormonal causes. Nutritional antioxidants (polyphenols) safeguard against dangerous lipoprotein (LDL) oxidation and atherosclerosis.

Bread and **cereals**, particularly whole wheat, provide protein, fiber, vitamins, minerals and energy without much fat. They add variety to meals, calm hunger, and help to keep caloric intake and obesity under control. The fibers that they contain help keep the intestine regular, reduce the risk of diverticulum inflammation and irritable bowel syndrome. Finally, soluble fibers contained in strawberries, oats, peas and legumes can contribute to lowering blood cholesterol.

Olive oil is the major source of fat in the Mediterranean diet. The monounsaturated fats, and to a lesser extent the polyunsaturated fats in olive oil, reduce total cholesterol blood levels without changing artery-friendly cholesterol levels (HDL). The monounsaturated fats and natural antioxidants in extra-virgin olive oil help prevent heart disease and stroke. In addition, monounsaturated oils protect against breast cancer and help keep arterial blood pressure low.

Fish and **lean meat** provide proteins needed for many vital functions as well as being important sources of vitamins and minerals. The polyunsaturated fats of the omega-3 series, found in fish such as mackerel and herring, help maintain the blood fluid (lower the risk of clotting) and prevent sudden death.

Cheese, **yogurt** and **milk**, eaten moderately, provide calcium, protein and vitamin B.

Wine taken at mealtimes in limited amounts (two glasses of red wine for a man and one glass for a woman) helps prevent atherosclerosis and alleviates stress by inhibiting adrenaline secretion.

Fresh foods guarantee low sodium content which is an important way to prevent arterial hypertension.

The people in Mediterranean countries living on a diet with the aforementioned characteristics have less heart disease than northern European populations. Moreover, this kind of diet helps protect against diabetes, obesity and some kinds of tumors. It has been estimated in fact that about 35% of all tumor-associated deaths may be attributed to dietary factors.

A healthy diet is part of a healthy lifestyle. Other habits to adopt in order to reap the maximum effect of a balanced diet are to exercise regularly (take a walk, bicycle, go swimming), avoid smoking, and make a conscious effort to relieve stress.

Limiting total fat intake to lower blood cholesterol levels in Mediterranean countries means eating less olive oil. This leads to less legume and vegetable consumption. By favoring mono- and polyunsaturated fatty acids over saturated fatty acids the low-fat diet developed by the American Heart Association comes ever closer to the Mediterranean diet.

The *Lyon Diet Heart Study* conducted in France on patients who had experienced one heart attack showed that a diet like the one eaten on Crete, with mostly monounsaturated fats (oleic acid) and omega-3 series polyunsaturated fatty acids (linolenic acid), better protects the cardiovascular system and causes fewer deaths than a diet rich in linoleic acid (omega-6 series polyunsaturated fatty acids) recommended for these same patients.

The *GISSI 4* (Italian study of post-infarction survival) recently showed that omega-3 series polyunsaturated fatty acid supplements (eicosapentaenoic and docosaesaenoic acids mostly present in fish) given to patients with coronary heart disease, protects the heart and lowers mortality by 21%.

A typical Mediterranean view.

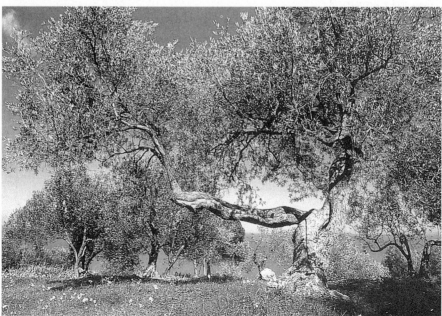

The diet of our ancestors living between 10,000-15,000 years ago was tightly hinged on availability of food from the hunt (meats) and gathering (vegetables). The term "hunter-gatherer" well defines this pattern. Such a diet had to provide enough fat to cover 20% of the daily energy needs, with saturated fats being 7-8%, polyunsaturated fats 5-6% and the remainder monounsaturated. The omega-6/omega-3 polyunsaturated fatty acid ratio was probably 4-3. In other words, for every molecule of omega-3 eaten, there were 3 or 4 omega-6 molecules. In real terms, the effects are difficult to determine. Studies indicate, however, that a diet rich in omega-6 at the expense of omega-3 increases the risk of heart disease.

The recent industrial revolution caused the first imbalance in these percentages. People ate more red meat and margarine (hydrogenated polyunsaturated fats). Subsequently, in the second half of the 20th century, the quantity of polyunsaturated vegetable oils, especially omega-6 series, steadily rose. This occurred because of the scientific evidence showing a drop in cholesterol levels associated with their use. At the same time, this happened at the expense of the omega-3 series of polyunsaturated fatty acids, which steadily fell. Currently the omega-6/omega-3 ratio in a Western society diet is about 15:1. It has more than tripled. It is possible that the omega-3 fatty acids adapted over this long period (but there has not been ample time for genetic change to occur) carry out essential functions that have in part balanced out the effects of excessive omega-6 fatty acids. According to this theory, the imbalance between these fundamental components of the cell membrane (more omega-6 than omega-3) is at least partially responsible for increased cardiovascular risk present in populations with a Western society diet.

The return to a traditional Mediterranean diet has now become a primary goal of many populations. The United States is waging a major campaign to lower cholesterol levels and increase vegetables in the diet. People are ready to change habits provided that the recommendations are positive. It is easier to be heeded when telling people what they should include in their diet to promote good heath than what they should avoid. The nutritional recommendations to prevent heart disease made by the American Heart Association were appropriate.

The most prudent and scientifically sound advice for the population at large is to eat a balanced diet rich in natural antioxidants contained in fruit, vegetables and whole grained cereals.

More recently (2001), the American Heart Association issues a scientific advisory statement that a Mediterranean-style diet demonstrates impressive effects on cardiovascular diesease. Accordingly, all should take advantage of the possible opportunity to dramatically lower cardiovascular disease risk (and perhaps cancer risk) in the population by widely recommending a diet that features a dietary pattern that includes fruits, root vegetables (carrots, turnips, potatoes, onions, radishes), leafy green vegetables, breads and cereales, fish, and foods high in oleic acid and α-linolenic acid such as vegetables oils (olive, flaxseed, canola), and nuts and seeds (walnuts and flaxseed).

Though we are already fully aware of what good health implies, how witty and wise were the following words by Mark Twain:

Health is much more than the absence of disease.

References

Chapter 1

ALLBAUGH L.G. *Crete, a case study of an underdeveloped area.* Princeton, NJ: Princeton University Press, 1953.

ATTENBOROUGH D. *Il primo paradiso. L'uomo e il mondo del Mediterraneo.* De Agostini, 1987.

NESTLE M. *Mediterranean diets: historical and research overview.* The American Journal of Clinical Nutrition 61: 1313S-1320S, 1995.

STRABONE. *Geografia (L'Italia), libri I-IV.* Rizzoli, 1988.

WILLETT W.C., SACKS F., TROCHOPOULOU A., et al. *Mediterranean diet pyramid: a cultural model for healthy eating.* The American Journal of Clinical Nutrition. 61: 1402S-1406S, 1995.

Chapter 2

AA.VV. *Viaggio nell'Egitto dei Faraoni.* De Agostini, 1985.

BRESCIANI E. *A pranzo nell'antico Egitto.* Archeo, De Agostini, 1985.

CURTO S., ROCCATI A. *Tesori dei Faraoni.* De Agostini, 1985.

ERODOTO. *Le Storie, libri I-II: Lidi, Persiani, Egizi.* Garzanti, 1989.

LECA A.-P. *La Medicina Egizia: Igiene alimentare.* Ciba-Geigy, 1986, pp. 302-312.

MEEKS D., FAVARD-MEEKS C. *La vita quotidiana degli egizi e dei loro dei.* BUR Rizzoli, 1995.

MONTET P. *La vita quotidiana in Egitto ai tempi di Ramses.* BUR Rizzoli, 1999.

SAUNERON S. *Villés et légendes d'Egypte.* Il Cairo, 1983.

TACCONI B. *Lo schiavo Hanis.* Oscar Mondadori, 1988.

WALTARI M. *Sinuhe l'egiziano.* Superbur Rizzoli, 1989.

Chapter 3

AA.VV. *I Fenici.* Bompiani, 1988.

AA.VV. *Sikanie: storia e civiltà della Sicilia greca.* Istituto Veneto di Arti Grafiche, 1985.

Bondì S.F. *L'alimentazione nell'antichità: l'alimentazione nel mondo fenicio-punico.* Parma, 1985, pp. 167-184.

Bondì S.F. *Pranzo a Cartagine.* Archeo, De Agostini, 1986.

Moscati S. *Cartagine, regina dei mari.* Archeo Dossier, De Agostini, Settembre 1985.

Moscati S. *Italia ricomparsa: preistorica, greca, fenicia.* Touring Club Italiano, 1983.

Chapter 4

AA.VV. *Eros Grec: Amour des Dieuxs et des Hommes.* Editions du Ministére de la Culture de Grèce, Direction des Antiquités. Atene, 1989.

Ateneo. *Schiavi e servi.* Sellerio, Palermo, 1990.

Athenee de Naucratis. *Les Deipnosophistes, livres I-II.* Les Belles Lettres, Paris, 1956.

Boardman J. *Athenian black figure vases.* Thames and Hudson, London, 1974.

Boardmam J. *La ceramica antica.* Mondadori, 1984.

D'Andria F. *I Greci in Italia.* Archeo Dossier n. 20, De Agostini.

Flaceliére R. *La vita quotidiana in Grecia nel secolo di Pericle.* BUR Rizzoli, 1987.

Higgins R. *Creta: la civiltà del Minotauro.* Newton Ragazzi, 1978.

Napoli M. *La tomba del tuffatore.* De Donato Editore, 1970.

Race G. *La cucina del mondo classico.* Edizioni Scientifiche Italiane, 1999.

Salles C. *I bassifondi dell'antichità.* BUR Rizzoli, 1984.

Salza Prina Ricotti E. *A pranzo nell'antica Grecia.* Archeo, De Agostini, 1985.

Vernant J.P. *L'uomo greco.* Laterza, 1999.

Chapter 5

AA.VV. *La ceramica degli Etruschi.* De Agostini, 1987.

Cristofani M. *Etruschi: cultura e società.* De Agostini, 1978.

Erodoto. *Le Storie, libri I-II, Lidi, Persiani ed Egizi.* Garzanti, 1989.

Giugliano D. *The obese Etruscan.* Journal of Endocrinological Investigation 24: 206; 2001.

Heurgeon J. *Vita quotidiana degli Etruschi.* Oscar Mondadori, 1998.

Moscati S. *Italia ricomparsa: etrusca, italica.* Touring Club Italiano, 1984.

Sassatelli G. *A pranzo con gli Etruschi.* Archeo, De Agostini, 1986.

Sterpellone L. *La medicina etrusca: usi e costumi alimentari.* Ciba-Geigy, 1990, pp. 81-106.

Torelli M. *Necropoli dell'Italia antica*. Touring Club Italiano, 1982.
Waltari M. *Turms l'etrusco*. BUR Rizzoli, 1987.

Chapter 6

AA.VV. *Il tesoro di Boscoreale*. Franco Maria Ricci, 1988.
AA.VV. *L'alimentazione nel mondo antico. I Romani: età imperiale*. Poligrafico e Zecca dello Stato, Roma, 1987.
AA.VV. *Pompei, abitare sotto il Vesuvio*. Ferrara Arte, 1996.
André J. *L'alimentation et la cuisine à Rome*. Les Belles Lettres, Parigi, 1981.
Apicio. *Manuale di gastronomia*. Rizzoli, 1967.
Bisconti F. *A pranzo con gli antichi cristiani*. Archeo, De Agostini, 1986.
Cantarella E., Iacobelli L. *Un giorno a Pompei: vita quotidiana, cultura, società*. Electa, Napoli, 1999.
Dosi A., Schnell F. *Le abitudini alimentari dei Romani*. Edizioni Quasar, Roma, 1992.
Dosi A. Schnell F. *I Romani in cucina*. Edizioni Quasar, Roma, 1992.
Etienne R. *La vita quotidiana a Pompei*. Milano, 1973.
Giovenale D.C. *Le Satire*. Einaudi, 1983.
Gozzini Giacosa I. *A cena da Lucullo*. Piemme, 1986.
Gozzini Giacosa I. *Mense e cibi della Roma antica*. Piemme, 1996.
Guerdan R. *Pompei: la vita di una città prima della morte*. Oscar Mondadori, 1978.
Maiuri A. *Pompei ed Ercolano: tra case ed abitanti*. Giunti, 1998.
Petronio Arbitro. *Satyricon*. Rizzoli, 1988.
Salza Prina Ricotti E. *A pranzo nell'antica Roma*. Archeo, De Agostini, 1986.
Salza Prina Ricotti E. *Ricette della cucina romana a Pompei e come eseguirle*. L'Erma di Bretschneider, Roma, 1993.
Staccioli R. *Pompei: la vita quotidiana*. Archeo Dossier, De Agostini, Agosto 1985.
Staccioli R. *Un giorno nell'antica Roma*. Archeo Dossier, De Agostini, Maggio 1985.
Valerio N. *La tavola degli antichi*. Mondadori, 1989.

Chapter 7

Billiard R. *La vigne dans l'antiquité*. Edition Lardanchet, Lyon, 1913.
Brillat-Savarin A. *Physiologie du goût*. Edition Hermann, Paris, 1975.
Cicirelli C. *Le ville rustiche*. In: *Pompei: abitare sotto il Vesuvio*, Ferrara Arte, 1997, pp. 29-33.

CICIRELLI C. *Attività Soprintendenza Terzigno.* Riv. St. Pomp. III, pp. 249-253; V, pp. 208-211; VI, pp. 228-239; VII, pp. 183-185.

DE CARO S. *La villa rustica in località Villa Regina di Boscoreale.* Roma, 1994.

DURRY M. *Les fammes et le vin.* Revue des Etudes Latines, T. XXXIII, 1956.

FERGOLA L, PAGANO M. *Oplontis.* Torre del Greco, 1998.

MANZON D. *Vini della Campania.* Ulisse & Calipso, Napoli, 1992.

MIELSCH H. *La villa romana.* Firenze, 1990.

TOHERNIA A. *Il vino: produzione e commercio.* In: Pompei 79, Napoli 1979, pp. 87-96.

Chapter 8

CAPURSO A., DE FANO S. *L'olio d'oliva: dal mito alla scienza.* CIC Edizioni Internazionali, Roma, 1998.

CORANDINI A. *La villa romana e la produzione schiavistica.* Storia di Roma, IV. Caratteri e Morfologia. Torino, 1989, pp. 101-192.

D'ARMS J.H. *Ville rustiche e ville di otium.* In: Pompei 79, Napoli 1979, pp. 65-87.

MACRÌ T., LA PORTA G., PICONE G. *Molise, terra d'olivo e d'olio.* Editrice Lampo, Campobasso, 1997.

PASQUI A. *La villa pompeiana della Pisanella presso Boscoreale.* Monum. Ant. Accad. Lincei, 1897.

Chapter 9

AA.VV. *Euphronios, Peintre à Athénes au VI siècle avant J.-C.* Réunion des Musées Nationaux, Paris, 1990.

BUSSAGLI M. *Il nudo nell'arte.* Giunti, 1998.

CARCOPINO J. *La vita quotidiana a Roma.* Laterza, 1999.

FLACELIÉRE R. *La vita quotidiana in Grecia nel secolo di Pericle.* BUR Rizzoli, 1987.

LA ROCCA E., DE VOS E., DE VOS A. *Guida archeologica di Pompei.* Mondadori, 1976.

LEVI M.A. *Roma antica.* Utet, Torino, 1963.

STACCIOLI R. *La civiltà di Roma.* Biblioteca di Storia patria, Roma, 1964.

WEYNE P. *Le pain et le cirque. Sociologie historique d'un pluralisme politique.* Le Seuil, Paris, 1976.

Chapter 10

ABELOW B.J., HOLFORD T.R., INSOGNA K.L. *Cross-cultural association between dietary animal proteins and hip fracture: a hypothesis.* Calcification Tissue Inter. 50: 14-18, 1992.

ALBERT C.M., HENNEKENS C.H., O'DONNELL C.J., et al. *Fish consumption and risk of sudden cardiac death.* The Journal of the American Medical Association 279: 23-28, 1998.

AUGUSTSSON K., et al. *Dietary heterocyclic amines and cancer of colon, rectum, bladder and kidney: a population-based study.* The Lancet 353: 703-707, 1999.

CANNON G. *Food and health: the experts agree.* London, Consumers' Association, 1992.

DE LORGERIL M., SALEN P., MARTIN J.-L., et al. *Mediterranean diet, traditional risk factors, and the rate of cardiovascular complications after myocardial infarction.* Circulation 99: 779-785, 1999.

DE SELLMEJER, et al. *A high ratio of dietary animal to vegetable protein increases the rate of bone loss and the risk of fracture in postmenopausal women.* The American Journal of Clinical Nutrition 73: 118-122, 2001.

HEGSTED D.M. *Calcium and osteoporosis.* Journal of Nutrition 116: 2316-2319, 1986.

KATAN M.B. *Are there good and bad carbohydrates for HDL-cholesterol?* The Lancet 353: 1029-1030, 1999.

KEY T.J., FRASER G.E., THOROGOOD M., et al. *Mortality in vegetarians and nonvegetarians: detailed findings from a collaborative analysis of 5 prospective studies.* The American Journal of Clinical Nutrition 70: 516S-524S, 1999.

LIU S., WILLETT W.C., STAMPFER M.J., et al. *A prospective study of dietary glycemic load, carbohydrate intake, and risk of coronary heart disease in US women.* The American Journal of Clinical Nutrition 71: 1455-1461, 2000.

LYRITIS G. *Epidemiology and socioeconomic cost of osteoporotic fractures in Greece.* Calcification Tissue Inter. 51: 93-94, 1992.

MOSS M., FREED D.L.J. *Survival trends, coronary event rates, and the MONICA project.* The Lancet 354: 862, 1999.

SNOWDON D.A., PHILLIPS R.L., FRASER G.E. *Meat consumption and fatal ischemic heart disease.* Preventive Medicine 13: 490-500, 1984.

US DEPARTMENT OF AGRICULTURE. *The food guide pyramid.* Hyattsville, MD: Human Nutrition Information Service, 1992.

WILLETT W.C. *The dietary pyramid: does the foundation needs repair?* The Americam Journal of Clinical Nutrition 68: 218-219, 1998.

WILLETT W.C. *Convergence of philosophy and science: the Third International Congress on Vegetarian Nutrition.* The Americam Journal of Clinical Nutrition 70: 434S-438S, 1999.

WOLK A., MANSON J.E., STAMPFER M.J., et. al. *Long-term effect of dietary fiber and decreased risk of coronary heart disease among women.* The Journal of the American Medical Association 281: 1988-2004, 1999.

WORLD CANCER RESEARCH FUND. *Food, nutrition and the prevention of cancer: a global perspective.* Washington, D.C.: American Institute for Cancer Research, 1997.

Chapter 11

AHMAD K. *Gentle weight training recommended for older hearts.* The Lancet 355: 629, 2000.

BOSTOM A.G., GARBER C. *Endpoints for homocysteine-lowering trials.* The Lancet 355: 511-512, 2000.

BYERS T. *Diet, colorectal adenomas, and colorectal cancer.* The New England Journal of Medicine 342: 1206-1207, 2000.

CAO Y., et al. *Angiogenesis is inhibited by drinking tea.* Nature 398: 381, 1999.

COOKE J.P. *Nutriceuticals for cardiovascular health.* The American Journal of Cardiology 82(10A): 43S-46S, 1998.

FEDELE D. *Vino e salute: il paradosso francese.* Medico & Metabolismo 2: 27-37, 1998.

FESKENS E.J.M. *Can diabetes be prevented by vegetable fat?.* Diabetes Care 24: 1517-1518, 2001.

FINKEL E. *Phyto-oestrogens: the way to postmenopausal health?* The Lancet 352: 1762, 1999.

GINSBURG J., PRELEVIC G.M. *Lack of significant hormonal effects and controlled trials on phyto-oestrogens.* The Lancet 335: 163-164, 2000.

GIUGLIANO D., MARFELLA R., COPPOLA L., et al. *Vascular effects of acute hyperglycemia in humans are reversed by L-arginine.* Circulation 95: 1783-1790, 1997.

GIUGLIANO D., CERIELLO A., PAOLISSO G. *Oxidative stress and diabetic vascular complications.* Diabetes Care 19, 257-267, 1996.

GIUGLIANO D. *Antioxidants alimentaires et santé: quel role, par quels mécanismes?* 40emes Journées Nationales de Diététique, Marseille, 21-25 Avril, 1999.

GIUGLIANO D. *Dietary antioxidants for cardiovascular prevention.* Nutrition, Metabolism and Cardiovascular Diseases 10: 38-44, 2000.

GIUGLIANO D. *Diet and risk of cancer.* 42emes Journées Nationales de Diétetique, Marseille, 5-7 Avril, 2001.

GIUGLIANO D. *Type 2 diabetes.* Medical Crossfire 3: 20-21, 2001.

GIUNTA R., BENCIVENGA G., CARRATURO N., GIUGLIANO F. *Breve storia dell'idrologia.* Medico & Metabolismo 3: 63-64, 1999.

GLASS T., et al. *Population based study of social and productive activities as predictors of survival among elderly americans.* British Medical Journal 319: 478-483, 1999.

GONÇA A., BOBAK M. *Albanian paradox, another example of protective effect of Mediterranean lifestyle.* The Lancet 350: 1815-1817, 1997.

HERTOG M.G.L., et al. *Dietary antioxidant flavonoids and risk of coronary heart disease: The Zutphen Elderly Study.* The Lancet 342: 1007-1011, 1993.

HOPE Study Investigators. *Vitamin E supplementation and cardiovascular events in high-risk patients.* The New England Journal of Medicine 345: 154-160, 2000.

HOOVER R.N. *Cancer – Nature, nurture, or both.* The New England Journal of Medicine 343: 135-136, 2000.

HU F.B., MANSON J.E., STAMPFER M.J., et al. *Diet, lifestyle, and the risk of type 2 diabetes mellitus in women.* The New England Journal of Medicine 345: 790-797, 2001.

HOWARD G., et al. *Cigarette smoking and progression of atherosclerosis.* The Journal of the American Medical Association 279: 119-124, 1998.

JACOB R.A., BURRI B.J. *Oxidative damage and defence.* The American Journal of Clinical Nutrition 63: 985S-990S, 1996.

JACQUES P.F., SELHUB J., BOSTOM A.G., et al. *The effect of folic acid fortification on plasma folate and total homocysteine concentrations.* The New England Journal of Medicine 340: 1449-1454, 1999.

JANG M., CAI L., UDEANI G.O., et al. *Cancer chemopreventive activity of resveratrol, a natural product derived from grapes.* Science 275: 218-220, 1997.

JOHNSTON P.K., SABATÉ J. (Eds). *Third International Congress on Vegetarian Nutrition.* The American Journal of Clinical Nutrition 70: 429S-634S, 1999.

KEYS A. *Seven countries: a multivariate analysis of death and coronary heart disease.* Cambridge: Harvard University Press, 1980.

KULLER L.H. *A time to stop prescribing antioxidant vitamins to present and treat heart disease?* Arteriosclerosis, Thrombosis, and Vascular Biology, 21: 1253; 2001.

LARKIN M. *Centenarians point the way to healthy ageing.* The Lancet 353: 1074, 1999.

LARKIN M. *Benefits of walking should be taken to heart.* The Lancet 354: 134, 1999.

LAW M., WALD N. *Why heart disease is low in France: the time lag explanation.* British Medical Journal 318: 1471-1480, 1999.

MALINOW M.R., BOSTOM A.G., KRAUSS R.M. *Homocyst(e)ine, diet and cardiovascular diseases.* Circulation 99: 178-182, 1999.

MARFELLA R., GIUGLIANO G., CICCARELLI P. *Attività fisica e salute.* Medico & Metabolismo 3: 91-95, 1999.

MCCULLY K.S. *Homocysteine and vascular disease.* Nature Medicine 2: 386-389, 1996.

NAPPO F., DE ROSA N., MARFELLA R., DE LUCIA D., INGROSSO D., PERNA A.F., FARZATI B., GIUGLIANO D. *Impairment of endothelial functions by acute hyperhomocysteinemia and reversal by antioxidant vitamins.* The Journal of the American Medical Association 281: 2113-2118, 1999.

NUTTAL S.L., KENDALL M.J., MARTIN V. *Antioxidant therapy for the prevention of cardiovascular disease.* Quarterly Journal of Medicine 92: 239-244, 1999.

OLSHANSKY S.J., CARNES B.A., DÉSESQUELLES A. *Prospects for human longevity.* Science 291: 1491-1492, 2001.

ORNISH D., et al. *Avoiding revascularization with lifestyle changes: The Multicenter Lifestyle Demonstration Project.* The American Journal of Cardiology 82(10B): 72T-76T, 1998.

PENDURTHI U.R., WILLIAMS J.T., RAOL V.M. *Resveratrol, a polyphenolic compound found in wine, inhibits tissue factor expression in vascular cells.* Arteriosclerosis Thrombosis Vascular Biology 19: 419-426, 1999.

POTTER J. *Fiber and colorectal cancer- where to now?* The New England Journal of Medicine 340: 223-224, 1999.

RIMM E.B., STAMPFER M.J. *The role of antioxidants in preventive cardiology.* Current Opinions in Cardiology 12: 188-194, 1997.

ROBERTSON R.M., SMAHA L. *Can a Mediterranean-style diet reduce heart disease?* Circulation 103: 1821-1822, 2001.

SALMERON J., HU F.B., MANSON J.E., et al. *Dietary fat intake and risk of type 2 diabetes in women.* The American Journal of Clinical Nutrition 73: 1019-1026, 2001.

SCHOLL J. *Doctor, is wine good for my heart?* The Lancet 354: 514, 1999.

SESSO H., et al. *More evidence that tea is good for the heart.* The Lancet 353: 384, 1999.

SIES H. *Antioxidants in Disease Mechanisms and Therapy.* San Diego, Academic, 1997.

ST. CLAIR R. *Cardiovascular effects of soybean phytoestrogens.* The American Journal of Cardiology 82(10A): 40S-42S, 1998.

STRONG J.P., MALCOM G.T., McMAHAN C.A., et al. *Prevalence and extent of atherosclerosis in adolescents and young adults: implications for prevention from the Pathobiological Determinants of Atherosclerosis in Youth Study.* The Journal of the American Medical Association 281: 727-735, 1999.

TJØNNELAND A., GRØNBOEK M., STRIPP C., OVERVAD K. *Wine intake and diet in a random sample of 48,763 Danish men and women.* The American Journal of Clinical Nutrition 69: 49-54, 1999.

TUOMILETHO J., LINDSTRÖM J., ERIKSSON J.G., et al. *Prevention of type 2 diabetes mellitus by changes in lifestyle among subjects with impaired glucose tolerance.* The New England Journal of Medicine 344: 1343-1350, 2001.

VAN DEN HOOGEN P.C.W., FESKENS E.J.M., NAGELKERKE N.J.D., et al. for the Seven Countries Study Research Group. *The relation between blood pressure and mortality due to coronary heart disease among men in different part of the world.* The New England Journal of Medicine 342: 1-8, 2000.

VINICK M. *Cancer and diet.* Nutrition, Metabolism and Cardiovascular Diseases 9, (Suppl.) 52-55, 1999.

VITA J.A., KEANEY J.F.JR. *Exercise - Toning up the endothelium?* The New England Journal of Medicine 342: 503-505, 2000.

WILLETT W.C. *Diet and health: what should we eat.* Science 264: 532-537, 1994.

YOUNG D.R., et al. *Tai Chi gently reduces blood pressure in elderly.* The Lancet 353: 904, 1999.

Chapter 12

GISSI-Prevenzione Investigators. *Dietary supplementation with n-3 polyunsaturated fatty acids and vitamin E after myocardial infarction.* The Lancet 354: 447-455, 1999.

GIUGLIANO D., NAPPO F., COPPOLA L. *Pizza and vegetables don't stick to the endothelium.* Circulation 104: 34-35, 2001.

HOLMES M., et al. *Association of dietary intake of fat and fatty acids with risk of breast cancer.* The Journal of the American Medical Association 281: 914-920, 1999.

HU F., et al. *A prospective study of egg consumption and risk of cardiovascular disease in men and women.* The Journal of the American Medical Association 281: 1387-1394, 1999.

KEYS A. *Mediterranean diet and public health: personal reflections.* The American Journal of Clinical Nutrition 61: 1321S-1323S, 1995.

KEYS A., FIDANZA F., SCARDI V., et al. *Studies on serum cholesterol and other characteristics on clinically healthy men in Naples.* Archives of Internal Medicine 93: 328-335, 1954.

KEYS A., KEYS M. *How to eat well and stay well: the Mediterranean way.* New York: Doubleday & Company, 1975.

KRIS-ETHERTON P., ECKEL R.H., HOWARD B.V., ST. JEOR S., BAZZARRE T.L. *Lyon Diet Heart Study. Benefits of a Mediterranean-style, national cholesterol education program/American Heart Association Step I dietary pattern on cardiovascular disease.* Circulation 103: 1823-1825, 2001.

KUSHI L.H., LENART E.B., WILLETT W.C. *Health implications of Mediterranean diets in light of contemporary knowledge. 1. Plant food and dairy products.* The American Journal of Clinical Nutrition 61: 1407S-1415S, 1995.

KUSHI L.H., LENART E.B., WILLETT W.C. *Health implications of Mediterranean diets in light of contemporary knowledge. 2. Meat, wine, fats and oils.* The American Journal of Clinical Nutrition 61: 1416S-1427S, 1995.

LEAF A. *Dietary prevention of coronary heart disease. The Lyon Heart Study.* Circulation 99: 733-735, 1999.

214 THE WAY THEY ATE

MOORE P. *Fatty acids mitigate depression and dementia.* The Lancet 353: 1682, 1999.

SIMOPOULOS A.P. *Essential fatty acids in health and chronic disease.* The Americam Journal of Clinical Nutrition 70: 560S-569S, 1999.

TRIBBLE D.L. *Antioxidant consumption and risk of coronary heart disease: emphasis on vitamin C, vitamin E, and beta-carotene.* Circulation 99: 591-595, 1999.

VALMADRID C.T., KLEIN R., MOSS S.E., et al. *Alcohol intake and the risk of coronary heart disease mortality in persons with adult-onset diabetes mellitus.* The Journal of the American Medical Association 282: 239-246, 1999.

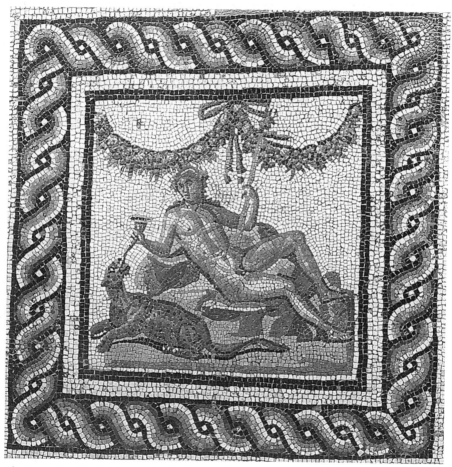

Floor mosaic of the triclinium in the domus of Villa Giulia at Brescia: a panther drinking from a horn offered by Dionysus.